BLOOD COLLECTION

FOURTH EDITION

400
Questions & Answers

Kathleen Becan-McBride, EdD, MT (ASCP)
Director, Community Outreach and Education
Coordinator, Texas-Mexico Border Health Services
Professor, School of Allied Health Sciences
Medical School—Dept. of Pathology & Laboratory Medicine
School of Public Health
School of Nursing
The University of Texas—Houston Health Science Center
Texas Medical Center, Houston, Texas

Assistant Director for Academic Partnerships
Greater Houston Area Health Education Center (AHEC)

Diana Garza, EdD, MT (ASCP), CLS (NCA)
Associate Professor, Department of Health Care Administration
College of Health Sciences, Texas Woman's University–Houston Center

Adjunct Associate Professor, Division of Laboratory Medicine
University of Texas M.D. Anderson Cancer Center
Houston, Texas

APPLETON & LANGE
Stamford, Connecticut

Notice: The authors and the publisher of this volume have taken care to make certain that the doses of drugs and schedules of treatment are correct and compatible with the standards generally accepted at the time of publication. Nevertheless, as new information becomes available, changes in treatment and in the use of drugs become necessary. The reader is advised to carefully consult the instruction and information material included in the package insert of each drug or therapeutic agent before administration. This advice is especially important when using, administering, or recommending new or infrequently used drugs. The authors and publisher disclaim all responsibility for any liability, loss, injury, or damage incurred as a consequence, directly or indirectly, of the use and application of any of the contents of this volume.

Copyright © 1998 by Appleton & Lange
A Simon & Schuster Company
Copyright © 1996, 1993, and 1989 by Appleton & Lange
Copyright © 1984 by Appleton-Century-Crofts

98 99 00 01 02 / 10 9 8 7 6 5 4 3 2 1

Prentice Hall International (UK) Limited, *London*
Prentice Hall of Australia Pty. Limited, *Sydney*
Prentice Hall Canada. Inc., *Toronto*
Prentice Hall Hispanoamericana, S.A., *Mexico*
Prentice Hall of India Private Limited, *New Delhi*
Prentice Hall of Japan, Inc., *Tokyo*
Simon & Schuster Asia Pte. Ltd., *Singapore*
Editora Prentice Hall do Brasil Ltda., *Rio de Janeiro*
Prentice Hall, *Upper Saddle River, New Jersey*

Library of Congress Cataloging-in-Publication Data
Becan-McBride, Kathleen, 1949-
    Phlebotomy/blood collection : 400 questions and answers / Kathleen
Becan-McBride, Diane Garza. — 4th ed.
        p.   cm. — (Appleton & Lange's quick review)
    Rev. ed. of: Phlebotomy examination review. 3rd ed. c1993.
    Sequenced and referenced to be used with: Phlebotomy handbook /
Diana Garza, Kathleen Becan-McBride. 4th ed. c1996.
    ISBN 0-8385-0334-9 (pbk. : alk. paper)
    1. Phlebotomy—Examinations, questions, etc. I. Garza, Diana
Phlebotomy handbook. II. Title. III. Series: A&L's quick review.
    [DNLM: 1. Blood Specimen Collection—examination questions.
    2. Phlebotomy—examination questions. QY 39 G245p 1998 Suppl.]
RB45.15.G37   1996 Suppl. 2
616.07'561—dc21
DNLM/DLC
for Library of Congress   97-30652

ISBN 0-8385-0334-9

Acquisitions Editor: Marinita Timban
Production Service: Inkwell Publishing Services
Production Editor: Lisa M. Guidone
Designer: Mary Skudlarek

PRINTED IN THE UNITED STATES OF AMERICA

*To my husband, Mark; my sons, Patrick and Jonathan;
my parents; my sister; and my parents-in-law
for their support and devotion.*

Kathleen Becan-McBride

*To my husband, Peter McLaughlin; my children,
Lauren, Kaitlin, and Kevin; and my parents
for their affection, patience, and constant support.*

Diana Garza

Contents

Preface

The quality of laboratory testing is dependent on the quality of the specimen obtained from the patient. Knowledge of proper technique and procedures in blood collection is the key to accurate and precise laboratory test results and subsequent diagnosis. The number of clinical laboratory tests and types of tests are increasing exponentially. This occurrence along with the addition of the managed health care environment have created new blood collection educational requirements and courses for various health care providers (e.g., phlebotomists, LVNs, RNs, medical technologists, medical assistants, physician care technicians, etc.). With the emphasis on knowledge and safety in blood collection, national board certification in phlebotomy has emerged and is required by many health care institutions, clinics, and physicians' offices as a result of federal, state, and quality assessment requirements. Because of these laws, continuing education in the practice of phlebotomy has become paramount.

These important events in phlebotomy served to shape this book, which is designed to act as a study companion for students who are (1) preparing for national board certification examinations and/or (2) pursuing self-assessment in phlebotomy.

Appleton & Lange's Quick Review: Phlebotomy/Blood Collection (Fourth Edition) enables the reader to review relevant material while becoming familiar with the types of questions given on board examinations. It is divided into *four* **comprehensive simulated examinations** consisting of 100 multiple-choice questions with referenced explanatory answers. The fourth edition incorporates up-to-date illustrations of blood collection equipment and techniques as bases for questions to help sharpen phlebotomy skills. Using this book will assist the reader in identifying areas of relative strength and weakness in the command of blood collection skills and responsibilities.

Some certification boards such as the ASCP Board of Registry administer the board examinations electronically. Therefore, a study disk is included to help prepare you for this computerized format. The review program includes the following key features:

- Diagnostic Exam helps assess your knowledge of each content area.
- Diagnostic Report identifies those topics that need further review and provides your overall score as well as a score for each content area.

Appleton & Lange's Quick Review: Phlebotomy/Blood Collection, Fourth Edition, and *Phlebotomy Handbook,* Fourth Edition, are major references for health care providers' educational programs, hospitals, physicians' offices, clinics, national examination boards, and legal issues in blood collection.

Introduction

History reveals that certification examinations for public responsibilities began in China thousands of years ago. The certification process in the United States has been and is currently required for many health care, legal, and public positions. The traditional method of measuring professional competence is the formal written examination. More recently, however, some certification boards have implemented computerized examinations.

Appleton & Lange's Quick Review: Phlebotomy/Blood Collection, Fourth Edition, is designed as a study aid to be used in preparation for the various phlebotomy certification examinations or as a means of self-assessment in phlebotomy. It provides a comprehensive review source, with *four* examinations of 100 multiple-choice questions each that are followed by answers and referenced explanations. Every question and answer is *content coded* to phlebotomy/blood collection subspecialty areas to help readers evaluate their areas of relative strength and weakness. These subspecialty areas with codes are as follows:

Subspecialty	Code
Blood Collection in Health Care Settings	HCS
Basic Anatomy and Physiology of Body Systems	AP
The Circulatory System	CS
Blood Collection Equipment	BCE
Venipuncture Procedures	VP
Skin Puncture Procedures	SPP
Complications in Blood Collection	CBC

Pediatric Phlebotomy	PP
Arterial and Special Collection Procedures	ASC
Home, Hospital Bedside, and Nursing Home Collections	HHB
Urinalysis and Body Fluid Collections	UBF
Infection Control	IC
Safety and First Aid	SFA
Specimen Documentation and Transportation	SDT
Total Quality Management	TQM
Communication, Professionalism, and Managerial Skills	CPM
Legal and Regulatory Issues	LRI
Appendices	AE

Study Strategy

In addition to having a sound knowledge base of phlebotomy topics, developing test-taking skills is important. Whether the national board examination is a written test or a computerized test, the examinee must have a discrete skill in answering multiple-choice questions, as well as the necessary phlebotomy skills. The first step in preparation for the examination is to schedule a specific period of time each week for studying the referenced material and answering the review questions. This time period should begin at least four to six months before the scheduled date of the examination. During the review of the topics, more time and effort should be directed toward the areas that are least familiar to the examinee. The number of topics to be reviewed should be totaled and divided by the number of weeks that are allowed for study. Then, the topics should be reviewed in one- to two-hour sessions per day during each week. For example, if 15 subspecialty topics in phlebotomy need to be reviewed prior to the examination and 16 weeks are allowed for the review, the examinee should study approximately one topic per week for approximately one hour per day for five days a week. Thus, two days a week can be allowed for rest.

During this review time, the examinee should thoroughly read the materials on the specific study topics in the *Phlebotomy Handbook,* and then take the first review examination in this book. Next, the examinee should check the answers at the end of the chapter and review the materials in the *Phlebotomy Handbook* if any of the answers are wrong. Software is included with *A&L's Quick Review* that allows each set of topics to be tested separately. This enables the reader to review an examination on those topics on which he or she needs more preparation. The questions on a particular topic should be retaken until all are answered correctly.

Phlebotomy Board Certification Organizations

Each of at least five organizations currently has board certification tests in phlebotomy. A reader intending to apply for one or more of the board examinations should determine which particular phlebotomy board certification examinations are better known and/or accepted in the local community and state. Following is a list of the major phlebotomy board certification organizations, their addresses, and their telephone numbers to assist in the application process:

American Society of Clinical Pathologists (ASCP)
Board of Registry
P.O. Box 12277
Chicago, IL 60612-0277
(312) 738-1336

American Medical Technologists (AMT)
710 Higgins Rd.
Park Ridge, IL 60068-5765
(847) 823-5169
(800) 275-1268

American Society of Phlebotomy Technicians (ASPT)
P.O. Box 1831
Hickory, NC 28603
(704) 322-1334

National Phlebotomy Association (NPA)
1901 Brightfeat Rd.
Landover, MD 20785
(301) 699-3846

National Certification Agency for Medical Laboratory Personnel (NCA)
P.O. Box 15945-289
Lenexa, KS 66285
(913) 438-5110

Taking the Examination

A good night's rest prior to the examination is recommended. It is also important to have a nutritious, but not heavy, meal prior to the examination. Tissues, cough drops, a wristwatch for timing questions, and other items necessary for personal comfort should be taken to the examination site. If allowed, a nutritious snack such as a granola bar might be taken for additional "brain" food.

The examination site must be located prior to the required examination time. One suggestion is to find the site and parking facilities the day before the examination. In addition, parking fee information should be obtained so that sufficient money can be taken along on the examination day. Identification materials, registration forms, and any other items required by the certification organization should also be taken along.

Allow plenty of time for travel to the examination site in case of unexpected mishaps such as traffic snarls. During travel, think positive thoughts (e.g., "My preparation for the exam was thorough, so I'll be able to answer the questions easily"). Maintain a confident attitude to prevent unnecessary stress.

After registration for the examination, allow time for reading the examination directions *thoroughly*. A calm, positive attitude is helpful during the necessary preliminary paperwork (e.g., filling out the answer sheet with name, examination type, and identification number). Before beginning the written examination, determine the amount of time that can be spent on each question. The examinee should never exceed the calculated time limit on the first attempt at each question. If a question is not answered within the allotted time period, it can be returned to after the other questions on the examination are completed. Usually, limited time is not a problem for the examinee during a written or computerized phlebotomy board examination.

During the examination, concentrate only on the questions at hand. All other matters, problems, and tasks should be placed in the back of the mind for consideration after the examination is complete. A wandering mind can be detrimental to test results!

Because some board examinations have different test sections with different question formats, it is important to be aware of changes in directions. Read each set of directions thoroughly before starting a new section of questions.

A helpful approach to selecting answers is to first read the stem of the question with *each* possible choice provided and eliminate choices that are obviously incorrect. Be cautious about choosing the first answer that *might* be correct; all possibilities should be considered before the final choice is made; the best answer should be selected. If a test booklet and a machine-scoreable answer sheet are being used, answers should be transferred to the answer sheet after a maximum of 20 questions are answered in the booklet. The answer sheet will be scored and *must* be filled out. Even though the correct answers may be written in the test booklet, credit will not be given unless these answers appear on the answer sheet. Make certain that the response next to the number on the answer sheet corresponds to the number in the test booklet!

If answers must be entered by means of computer, check the computer screen after an answer is entered to verify that the answer appears as it was entered.

The most important points to keep in mind during the examination are:

1. Keep a positive, confident attitude.

2. Stay calm and do the best possible.

3. Concentrate as much as possible during the examination.

Good luck! Now for the review examinations.

Practice Test Questions 1

DIRECTIONS (Questions 1–27): Each of the questions or incomplete statements below is followed by suggested answers or completions. Select the **BEST** answer in each case.

HCS

1. Which of the following hospital departments requires the use of heat, cold, water exercise, ultrasound or electricity, and other physical techniques to restore the patient's activity?

    A. Radiology
    B. Occupational therapy
    C. Radiation therapy
    D. Physical therapy

BCE

2. Which of the following anticoagulants is found in a light-blue-topped vacuum collection tube?

    A. EDTA
    B. Sodium heparin
    C. Sodium citrate
    D. Ammonium oxalate

CBC 3. A basal state exists

  A. after the evening meal
  B. before lunch
  C. 3 hr. after lunch
  D. in the early morning, 12 hr. after the last ingestion of food

PP 4. What needle gauge is required for scalp vein venipuncture of an infant?

  A. 17
  B. 19
  C. 21
  D. 23

ASC 5. In arterial blood gas collections, the needle should enter the artery at an angle of no less than

  A. 5°
  B. 15°
  C. 30°
  D. 45°

HHB 6. In terms of quality control procedures, SD stands for

  A. short distance
  B. standard deviation
  C. shared diameter
  D. standard dimension

UBF 7. Which of the following types of urine specimen is the "cleanest," or least contaminated?

  A. First morning specimen
  B. Timed specimen
  C. Midstream specimen
  D. Random specimen

IC **8.** Which of the following causes 40% of all nosocomial infections?

    A. Skin infections
    B. Wound infections
    C. Respiratory infections
    D. Urinary tract infections

SFA **9.** The first step in controlling severe bleeding is to

    A. send for medical assistance
    B. start cardiopulmonary resuscitation
    C. apply pressure directly over the wound or venipuncture site
    D. make the individual lie down and apply pressure to the person's forehead

LRI **10.** When a health care provider gives aid at an accident, he/she is usually protected through

    A. informed consent
    B. implied consent
    C. CPR law
    D. Rightful Action consent

AP **11.** Which of the following body systems allows carbon dioxide (CO_2) and oxygen (O_2) exchange?

    A. Nervous
    B. Muscular
    C. Respiratory
    D. Reproductive

CS   **12.** What happens to any region of the body that is deprived of blood for more than a few minutes?

      A. It dies
      B. It shrinks
      C. It makes the heart pump faster
      D. It makes a person breathe harder

VP   **13.** Where should the tourniquet be placed on the patient during the venipuncture procedure?

      A. 1 in. above the venipuncture
      B. Over the venipuncture site
      C. 3 in. above the venipuncture site
      D. 3 in. below the venipuncture site

SPP   **14.** Skin puncture **CANNOT** be used for which of the following tests?

      A. Glucose screening tests
      B. Coagulation studies
      C. CBC count and differential
      D. Cholesterol screening

SDT   **15.** The patient's medical record is

      A. the legal document that provides a chronological log of care
      B. the legal document that is available only to the patient's physician
      C. the procedure for a selected care plan
      D. public information that may be disclosed during a financial inquiry

TQM **16.** Dr. Avedis Donabedian pinpointed key aspects of health care functions that needed to be monitored for quality improvement. These functions included which of the following?

    A. Hematology instrumentation
    B. Structure, process, and outcomes
    C. Phlebotomy instrumentation
    D. Communication technology

CPM **17.** A patient's identity can best be confirmed by which of the following questions or statements?

    A. Are you Mr. Smith?
    B. Nurse Lauren said that you are Mr. Smith, so it must be true.
    C. What is your name?
    D. Please state your address.

LRI **18.** Examining witnesses before trial is referred to as

    A. discovery
    B. informed consent
    C. respondeat superior
    D. implied consent

HCS **19.** Of the following personnel, which health care worker is sometimes referred to as a *clinical laboratory technician*?

    A. Medical technologist
    B. Phlebotomist
    C. Medical laboratory technician
    D. Clinical laboratory scientist

AP   **20.** Which of the following body systems is the primary regulator of hormones?

      A. Digestive
      B. Endocrine
      C. Urinary
      D. Integumentary

CS   **21.** Leukocytes are

      A. red blood cells
      B. white blood cells
      C. platelets
      D. sera

BCE   **22.** If a blood specimen is allowed to clot, the result is

      A. plasma plus blood cells
      B. serum plus blood cells
      C. anticoagulated blood
      D. serum plus plasma

VP   **23.** The most important information on the patient's identification bracelet that can be used as sole confirmation for identification purposes is the patient's

      A. name
      B. hospital identification number
      C. room number and bed assignment, and the physician's name
      D. address and telephone number

SPP   **24.** Skin puncture blood is composed of

        A. venous blood
        B. arterial blood
        C. venous blood mixed with interstitial fluid
        D. blood from arterioles, venules, and capillaries, as well as interstitial fluid

CBC   **25.** Which of the following should stop the health care worker from collecting blood from a patient's arm vein?

        A. High blood pressure
        B. Mastectomy
        C. Heart attack that occurred 3 days ago
        D. Recent cardiac bypass surgery

PP   **26.** A commonly inherited disease detected through a blood screening process in neonates is

        A. phenylketonuria
        B. spina bifida
        C. neurogenic bladder abnormality
        D. carcinoma

ASC   **27.** Which artery is most frequently used for blood collection for arterial blood gas analysis?

        A. Radial
        B. Median cubital
        C. Brachial
        D. Femoral

DIRECTIONS (Questions 28–50): For each of the following questions or incomplete statements, **ONE** or **MORE** of the numbered responses are correct. In each case, select

A. if only 1, 2, and 3 are correct
B. if only 1 and 3 are correct
C. if only 2 and 4 are correct
D. if only 4 is correct
E. if all are correct

HHB   **28.** Which of the following statements is (are) true concerning Figure 1-1?

1. On day 10, the glucose control had a mean value of 100 mg/dL
2. On day 8, the glucose control was out of the ± 2 standard deviation level
3. On day 2, the glucose control read 103 mg/dL
4. On day 5, the glucose control was the same as the patient's glucose value

UBF   **29.** When a clean-catch urine specimen is needed, the health care worker should explain which of the following to a female patient?

1. The woman should squeeze the skin folds together around the urinary opening
2. The skin folds around the urinary opening should be cleaned with mild antiseptic soap and water
3. After collection, the urine specimen should be placed in a freezer until the analysis is performed
4. If the specimen is collected before the visit to the physician's office, the patient should label the container with her name and the time of collection

QUALITY CONTROL RECORD						TRIPPER HEALTH CARE INC.			

Instrument *Glucose Meter - Institution # 354*

Control Name and Lot # *Whole Blood Glucose Control Lot # 521*   Expiration Date: *8/24/95*

Supervisor Signature/Date:

TEST: *Glucose*   Units: *mg/dll*

Lower Limit *91*   Mean *100*   Upper Limit *109*

Date	No.	Value	Tech	Comment	Date	No.	Value	Tech	Comment
4/24/95	1	99	KBhu			17			
4/25/95	2	103	KBhu	prev. maintnan.		18			
4/26/95	3	100	KBhu			19			
4/27/95	4	100	KBhu			20			
4/28/95	5	105	KBhu	new battery		21			
4/29/95	6	97	KBhu			22			
4/30/95	7	95	KBhu			23			
5/1/95	8	96	KBhu			24			
5/2/95	9	103	KBhu			25			
5/3/95	10	100	KBhu			26			
5/4/95	11	103	KBhu			27			
5/5/95	12	97	KBhu			28			
	13					29			
	14					30			
	15					31			
	16								

Figure 1-1 Quality control record.

IC   **30.** Antiseptics for skin include(s)

1. ethyl alcohol
2. isopropyl alcohol
3. chlorhexidine
4. hexylresorcinol

SFA   **31.** If a fire occurs in or near electrical equipment, which of the following types of fire extinguishers should be used?

1. ABC
2. Class A
3. Class C
4. Class B

SDT   **32.** PROs use documentation in the medical records to

1. evaluate the quality of care
2. check for unnecessary procedures and tests
3. check the medical stability of patients
4. evaluate whether the patient's charges are warranted

TQM   **33.** Most clinical laboratories have written procedures about the inability to draw specimens. The procedure should cover which of the following circumstances?

1. Unsuccessful collection attempts
2. Patient unavailability
3. Patient refusal to have blood collected
4. Physicians' interference with the blood collection process

CPM   **34.** For the glucose tolerance test, the patient must

        1. remain fasting
        2. drink enough water to provide the timed urine specimens
        3. be available at specified times
        4. remain seated at all times during the test

LRI   **35.** The court systems (federal and state) generally have which of the following levels?

        1. Trial courts
        2. Intermediate courts
        3. Supreme courts
        4. Night courts

HCS   **36.** In which department(s) are high-energy x-rays, cobalt, and other types of radiation applied in the treatment of disease, especially cancer?

        1. Nuclear medicine
        2. Physical therapy
        3. Radiology
        4. Radiation therapy

HCS   **37.** The medical technologist is sometimes referred to as a

        1. MT
        2. CLS
        3. clinical laboratory scientist
        4. MTL

BCE **38.** Which of the following is (are) capillary blood collection system(s)?

1. Microvette
2. Unopette
3. Microtainer
4. Microtome

VP **39.** Identification of an inpatient can **BEST** be accomplished by matching the name on the requisition form with the

1. identification number on the hospital bracelet
2. hospital room number
3. patient's verbal statement of his/her name
4. patient's bed assignment

BCE **40.** Specimens for which of the following assays are frequently collected in gray-topped blood collection vacuum tubes?

1. Fasting blood glucose
2. Glucose
3. FBS
4. Glucose-6-phosphate dehydrogenase

BCE **41.** Specimens for which of the following tests must be collected in blue-topped blood collection tubes?

1. RVV time
2. Russell viper venom time
3. Stypven time
4. VDRL test

CBC **42.** Which of the following will cause changes in a basal state?

  1. Tourniquet application
  2. Stress and drugs
  3. Exercise
  4. Diet

ASC **43.** A prolonged bleeding time for a patient may be caused by the patient's intake of

  1. aspirin
  2. mithramycin
  3. ethyl alcohol
  4. dextran

PP **44.** The dorsal hand vein technique for infants includes which of the following steps?

  1. The patient's wrist veins are used
  2. The health care provider collecting the sample makes a tourniquet with his/her fingers
  3. The infant is stuck with a safety lancet
  4. Blood is collected directly from the hub of the needle

ASC **45.** Which of the following items is (are) needed to collect a blood culture specimen?

  1. Disposable gloves
  2. Iodine scrub swab stick
  3. Alcohol preps
  4. Four light-blue-topped blood collection tubes

HHB   **46.** Which of the following abbreviations refer(s) to the term *hematocrit?*

        1. Hct
        2. PCV
        3. Crit
        4. Hem

IC   **47.** A health care employee with which of the following diseases must avoid patient contact by not working until the disease is noninfectious?

        1. Hepatitis B
        2. Impetigo
        3. Chicken pox
        4. Rubella

BCE   **48.** Which of the following blood analytes is (are) sensitive to light?

        1. Lead
        2. Iron
        3. Calcium
        4. Bilirubin

AP   **49.** Bones are categorized into which of the following groups?

        1. Flat
        2. Long
        3. Irregular
        4. Short

HCS **50.** Which of the following exemplifies health care facilities in which blood collection is most likely to occur?

    1. Medical group practice
    2. HMO
    3. Multiphasic screening center
    4. Community health center

DIRECTIONS (Questions 51–100): Each of the questions or incomplete statements below is followed by suggested answers or completions. Select the **BEST** answer in each case.

AP **51.** How many chromosomes are contained in human cells?

    A. 25
    B. 50
    C. 46
    D. 106

TQM **52.** The JCAHO uses which of the following strategies for quality assessment of health care performance?

    A. A manufacturing model
    B. A phlebotomy model
    C. A modified Donabedian model
    D. A 10-step model

AE **53.** How do you state the phrase "I need to take a blood sample" in Spanish?

    A. Necesito sacar sangre
    B. Le va a doler un poquito
    C. Necesito picarle su dedo
    D. Como se llama?

BCE   **54.** If the phlebotomist collects only venipuncture specimens, which of the following items would **NOT** be needed on his/her specimen collection tray?

    A. Alcohol, iodine, and Betadine pads
    B. Disposable gloves
    C. Autolet II Clinisafe
    D. Tourniquet

VP   **55.** The term *stat* refers to

    A. abstaining from food for a period of time
    B. using timed blood collections for specific specimens
    C. using the early morning specimens for laboratory testing
    D. immediate and urgent specimen collection

CBC   **56.** An abnormal accumulation of fluid in the intercellular spaces of the body is

    A. petechia
    B. a thrombus
    C. a fomite
    D. edema

AP   **57.** The digestive system functions include which of the following?

    A. To break down food chemically and physically into nutrients
    B. Absorb nutrients to be used by body cells
    C. To eliminate the waste products of digestion
    D. All of the above

HCS **58.** The section of the clinical laboratory that tests for genetic fingerprinting is called the section of

    A. geriatrics
    B. blood banking
    C. clinical virology
    D. deoxyribonucleic acid probe analysis

SPP **59.** The average depth of a skin puncture on an adult should be

    A. 0.5–1.0 mm
    B. 2–3 mm
    C. 3–5 mm
    D. 2–3 cm

ASC **60.** A CVC is a

    A. central venous catheter
    B. control venous catheter
    C. central venous culture
    D. control venous corticosteroid

PP **61.** Which of the following childhood age groups is depicted by the following concerns: actively involved in anything concerning the body, embarrassed to show fear, and may act hostile to mask fear?

    A. Infants and toddlers
    B. Preschoolers
    C. School-age children
    D. Teenagers

AP   **62.** Meninges are defined as

    A. the causative agent of meningitis
    B. protective membrane coverings of the brain and spinal cord
    C. nerve impulses that transmit sensory functions
    D. cranial nerves

ASC   **63.** Which of the following tubes is used to collect specimens for blood culture determinations?

    A. Yellow-topped SPS tubes
    B. Yellow-topped ACD tubes
    C. Speckled-topped SST tubes
    D. Royal-blue-topped tubes

CPM   **64.** When a patient requests information about why a certain laboratory test was ordered, the health care worker should

    A. inform the patient about the test to the best of his/her knowledge
    B. ask the physical therapist to inform the patient
    C. not provide the information but refer the patient to the attending physician
    D. provide written information to the patient

LRI   **65.** If a physician orders laboratory tests for diagnosis and the patient comes to the laboratory with a rolled-up sleeve, he/she is giving

    A. implied consent
    B. informed consent
    C. Rightful Action consent
    D. preventive consent

AP   **66.** Which organ secretes bile?

        A. Pancreas
        B. Stomach
        C. Appendix
        D. Liver

HCS   **67.** Diagnosis and treatment of disorders and disabilities of the neuromuscular system are the functions of which department?

        A. Plastic surgery
        B. Physical medicine
        C. Geriatrics
        D. Radiology

ASC   **68.** To help minimize the incidence of dizziness, fainting, or other reactions to blood loss, blood donors are encouraged to eat within how many hours of donating blood?

        A. 9
        B. 8
        C. 7
        D. 6

HHB   **69.** Which of the following is released from the pancreas and has a major effect on blood glucose levels?

        A. ACTH
        B. Insulin
        C. Aldosterone
        D. Renin

AP   **70.** Glomeruli are best described as

        A. filters of the kidneys
        B. cells in the liver
        C. part of the digestive system
        D. part of the endocrine system

PP   **71.** When a skin puncture is performed on an infant or a child, which of the following specimens is collected first?

        A. Blood bank specimens
        B. Chemistry specimens
        C. Cytogenetic specimens
        D. Hematology specimens

ASC   **72.** Which of the following procedures requires 10 mL of normal saline and two or three 20-mL disposable syringes?

        A. Sweat chloride procedure
        B. Skin test for allergies
        C. Blood collection from a blood donor
        D. Blood collection through CVCs

UBF   **73.** Peritoneal fluid is located

        A. around the lungs
        B. in the joints
        C. in the abdomen
        D. in the sac around the heart

AP   **74.** The endocrine system can best be evaluated by

        A. a tissue biopsy
        B. analyzing hormone levels
        C. doing blood gas analysis
        D. testing spinal fluid

CS   **75.** Erythrocytes are

       A. red blood cells
       B. white blood cells
       C. platelets
       D. sera

BCE   **76.** Chromosome analysis requires whole blood collected in a

       A. green-topped tube
       B. serum-separator tube
       C. gray-topped tube
       D. light-blue-topped tube

VP   **77.** During venipuncture, the needle should be inserted at what angle to the skin?

       A. 5°
       B. 15°
       C. 45°
       D. 90°

HCS   **78.** In which of the following laboratory sections are personnel involved in the preparation and processing of tissue samples removed during surgery, autopsy, or other medical procedures?

       A. Clinical immunology
       B. Histology
       C. Transfusion medicine
       D. Clinical microbiology

AP **79.** Physiology is the study of

A. the functional components of the body
B. the mechanical makeup of the body
C. the structural components of the body
D. anabolic and catabolic mechanisms in the body

CBC **80.** Solid masses derived from blood constituents that reside in the blood vessels are

A. lymphocytes
B. thrombi
C. petechiae
D. fomites

ASC **81.** Which of the following specimens requires the use of a specially prepared acid-washed plastic syringe when the specimen is collected in a syringe?

A. Blood culture
B. Blood gases
C. Thyroxine
D. Trace elements

HHB **82.** Na^+, K^+, Cl^-, and HCO^-_3 are usually referred to as

A. electrolytes
B. blood gases
C. coagulation factors
D. endocrine hormones

IC   **83.** Which of the following is a commonly identified causative agent of nosocomial infections in a nursery unit?

     A. *Escherichia coli*
     B. *Haemophilus vaginalis*
     C. *Bordatella pertussis*
     D. *Vibrio cholerae*

AE   **84.** One meter is equivalent to

     A. 36 in.
     B. 39.37 in.
     C. 50.24 in.
     D. 55.8 in.

LRI   **85.** Before a patient's laboratory test results can legally be released, the patient must

     A. express verbal permission
     B. tell his/her doctor that it is okay
     C. provide written consent
     D. provide his/her lawyer's consent

TQM   **86.** Customer satisfaction is defined as meeting the needs of

     A. those who are being served
     B. physicians
     C. the JCAHO
     D. those who pay the bills

SDT **87.** Bar codes can be used in health care for patient identification purposes. Which of the following characterizes how bar codes are interpreted?

    A. They indicate prices for each of the laboratory procedures performed
    B. Light and dark bands of varying widths represent alphanumeric symbols
    C. They contain the name of the instrument
    D. They reveal if the proper mix of blood and additive has occurred as related to body weight

SFA **88.** If an accident occurs, such as a needle stick, what should the injured health care provider do first?

    A. Contact his/her immediate supervisor
    B. Fill out the necessary health care forms
    C. Cleanse the area with isopropyl alcohol and apply a Band-Aid
    D. Take the needle back to the clinical laboratory for verification of the accident

IC **89.** Which of the following chemical compounds is an antiseptic for skin?

    A. 1% phenol
    B. Hexachorophene
    C. Chlorophenol
    D. Ethylene oxide

UBF **90.** A 24-hr. urine specimen is usually collected to test for

    A. hormones
    B. therapeutic drug levels
    C. creatine kinase
    D. bacteria

ASC   **91.** Therapeutic phlebotomy is used in the treatment of

        A. iron-deficiency anemia
        B. chronic anemia
        C. megaloblastic anemia
        D. polycythemia

CBC   **92.** Tylenol (acetaminophen) use can lead to

        A. falsely increased values in skeletal muscle enzyme assays
        B. falsely increased values in liver function tests
        C. falsely decreased values in liver function tests
        D. falsely decreased values in skeletal muscle enzyme assays

SPP   **93.** Excessive massaging or milking of the finger during a skin puncture procedure may result in

        A. an adequate supply of blood to fill several capillary tubes
        B. increased venous blood flow to the puncture site
        C. hemolysis and contamination of the specimen with tissue fluid
        D. helpful results in glucose screening tests

VP   **94.** Which of the following information is essential for labeling a patient's specimen?

        A. Patient's name and identification number, date of collection, patient's room number, phlebotomist's initials
        B. Patient's name and identification number, date of collection, time of collection
        C. Patient's name and identification number, date and time of collection, phlebotomist's initials
        D. Patient's name and identification number, date of collection, physician's name

BCE   **95.** Which of the following anticoagulants is found in a green-topped blood collection vacuum tube?

A. Sodium polyanetholesulfonate
B. Sodium heparin
C. Sodium citrate
D. Ammonium oxalate

CS   **96.** Thrombocytes are

A. red blood cells
B. white blood cells
C. platelets
D. sera

AP   **97.** Which structure governs the functions of the individual cell, such as growth, repair, reproduction, and metabolism?

A. Membrane
B. Cytoplasm
C. Lysosome
D. Nucleus

HCS   **98.** Ionizing radiation for treating disease and fluoroscopic and radiographic x-ray instrumentation is used in what hospital department?

A. Occupational therapy
B. Physical therapy
C. Clinical laboratory
D. Radiology/medical imaging

AP   **99.** As CO_2 levels increase in the blood, the blood pH

   A. decreases
   B. increases
   C. stays the same
   D. increases for the first few minutes then drops to normal

AE   **100.** One gallon is equivalent to

   A. 5 L
   B. 4 L
   C. 3.78 L
   D. 2.72 L

Practice Test Questions 1

Answers and Discussion

Page numbers refer to Garza D, Becan-McBride K: *Phlebotomy Handbook, 4th ed.* Stamford, CT, Appleton & Lange, 1996.

1. **(D)** The role of the physical therapy department is to eliminate the patient's disability or to restore, as completely as possible, his/her mental or physical abilities. *(p. 15)*

2. **(C)** Sodium citrate is found in a light-blue-topped vacuum collection tube. *(p. 122)*

3. **(D)** A basal state exists in the early morning, 12 hr. after the last ingestion of food. *(p. 210)*

4. **(D)** A 23-gauge winged infusion set (butterfly needle) is required for scalp vein venipuncture of an infant. *(p. 249)*

5. **(D)** In arterial blood gas collections, the needle should enter the artery at an angle of no less than 45°. *(p. 264)*

6. **(B)** *SD* stands for *standard deviation*. *(p. 310)*

7. **(C)** The midstream, or clean-catch specimen, is the "cleanest" or least contaminated urine specimen. *(p. 325)*

8. **(D)** Urinary tract infections have a 40% prevalence rate of nosocomial infection. *(p. 345)*

9. **(C)** The first step in controlling severe bleeding is to apply pressure directly over the wound or venipuncture. *(pp. 392–393)*

10. **(B)** Implied consent exists when immediate action is required to save a patient's life. *(p. 499)*

11. **(C)** The respiratory system is involved in carbon dioxide (CO_2) and oxygen (O_2) exchange. *(p. 53)*

12. **(A)** Any region that is deprived of blood (carrying oxygen) will die after a few minutes. *(p. 72)*

13. **(C)** A tourniquet should be applied about 3 in. above the venipuncture site. *(p. 170)*

14. **(B)** Skin puncture blood should *not* be used for coagulation studies, blood cultures, and erythrocyte sedimentation rate (ESR) determinations. Sometimes, skin puncture cannot be used because testing may require larger amounts of blood (for blood cultures), interstitial fluids dilute the blood to some extent, and/or a patient has poor peripheral circulation. *(p. 194)*

15. **(A)** The medical record is the definitive legal document that provides a chronological log of the patient's care. *(p. 402)*

16. **(B)** Avedis Donabedian, a physician, pinpointed key aspects of health care functions that needed to be monitored for quality improvement. These functions included structure, process, and outcomes of health care services. *(p. 446)*

17. **(C)** A patient's identity can best be confirmed by asking the patient, "What is your name?" *(p. 467)*

18. **(A)** Examining witnesses before trial is referred to as *discovery.* *(p. 502)*

19. **(C)** The medical laboratory technician (MLT) is also referred to as a *clinical laboratory technician* (CLT). *(p. 21)*

20. (B) The endocrine system is the primary regulator of hormones. *(p. 62)*

21. (B) Leukocytes are white blood cells. *(p. 73)*

22. (B) If a blood specimen is allowed to clot, the result is serum plus blood cells meshed in a fibrin clot. *(pp. 79, 103)*

23. (B) The most important information on the patient's identification bracelet that can be used as sole confirmation for identification purposes is the patient's hospital identification number. *(p. 157)*

24. (D) The composition of skin puncture blood is significantly different from that of venous blood acquired by venipuncture. It is composed of blood from arterioles, venules, and capillaries, as well as some interstitial (tissue) fluid, which is released during the sticking process. *(p. 194)*

25. (B) A mastectomy (removal of a breast) can cause lymphostasis (no lymph flow) on that side of the body. Thus, a venipuncture must not be performed on the arm on the same side as the mastectomy since the patient is highly susceptible to infection. *(p. 207)*

26. (A) A commonly inherited disease detected through the blood screening process is phenylketonuria. *(pp. 241, 244)*

27. (A) The radial artery is most frequently used for blood collection for arterial blood gas analysis. *(p. 259)*

28. (B) Per Figure 1-1, the glucose control had a mean value of 100 mg/dL on day 10, and on day 2, the glucose control read 103 mg/dL. *(pp. 309–310)*

29. (C) When a clean-catch specimen is needed, the health care worker should explain to the female patient that the skin folds around the urinary opening should be cleaned with mild antiseptic soap and water, and that if the specimen is collected before the visit to the physician's office, the patient should label the container with her name and the time of the collection. *(p. 325)*

30. (E) Ethyl alcohol, isopropyl alcohol, chlorhexidine, and hexylresorcinol are antiseptics for skin use. *(p. 372)*

31. (B) If a fire occurs in or near electrical equipment, a multipurpose (ABC) or class C extinguisher can be used. *(p. 385)*

32. (E) PROs use documentation in the medical records to evaluate the quality of care, medical stability of patients, necessity of tests and procedures, adequacy of discharge planning, and occurrence of avoidable discomfort or death. PROs can impose fines, impose sanctions, or deny reimbursement for care if patient care is inappropriate. *(p. 404)*

33. (A) Most clinical laboratories have written procedures about the inability to draw specimens. The procedures usually cover what to do in the following circumstances: unsuccessful collection attempts, patient unavailability, and patient refusal to have blood collected. *(p. 460)*

34. (A) For the glucose tolerance test, the patient must remain fasting, drink enough water to provide the timed urine specimens, and be available at specified times for specimen collections. *(p. 468)*

35. (A) The court systems (federal and state) generally have trial, intermediate, and supreme courts. *(p. 493)*

36. (D) In the radiation therapy department, high-energy x-rays, cobalt, elution, and other types of radiation are applied in the treatment of disease, especially cancer. *(p. 14)*

37. (A) The medical technologist is sometimes referred to as an *MT* or a *clinical laboratory scientist,* which is abbreviated *CLS. (p. 20)*

38. (A) Capillary blood collection systems include the Microvette capillary blood collection system (Sarsedt Inc., Princeton, NJ), the B-D Unopette (Becton Dickinson and Co., Franklin Lakes, NJ), and the B-D Microtainer (Becton Dickinson VACUTAINER Systems and Co.). *(pp. 142–143)*

39. (B) Patient identification can best be accomplished by a three-way match among the patient's requisition form, the patient's identification bracelet or armband, and verbal statement of his/her name. Room numbers and hospital bed numbers should not be used to identify a patient because patients are frequently moved from one room or bed to another or are discharged and replaced by other patients. *(pp. 157, 159)*

40. **(A)**   FBS, fasting blood glucose, and glucose are the same assay; thus, all specimens for the assay are collected in gray-topped vacuum tubes. *(pp. 114–115)*

41. **(A)**   Russell viper venom time, also expressed as *RVV* or *Stypven time,* is an assay run on plasma collected in a blue-topped blood collection tube. *(p. 119)*

42. **(E)**   Tourniquet application, stress, drugs, exercise, and diet are among many factors that cause changes in the basal state and interfere with laboratory test results. *(p. 210)*

43. **(E)**   The intake of any of the following drugs can lead to a prolonged bleeding time: aspirin, mithramycin, ethyl alcohol, and dextran. *(pp. 268–269)*

44. **(C)**   For the dorsal hand vein technique for infants, the health care provider collecting the sample makes a tourniquet with his/her fingers and blood is collected directly from the hub of the needle. *(pp. 247–248)*

45. **(A)**   Disposable gloves, an iodine scrub swab stick (10% povidone-iodine solution with lathering agents), and alcohol preps are some of the items needed during collection of a blood culture specimen. *(p. 270)*

46. **(A)**   *Hct, PCV,* and *Crit* are all abbreviations for the term *hematocrit. (p. 315)*

47. **(E)**   If an employee of a health care institution has hepatitis B, impetigo, chicken pox, or rubella, he/she cannot work at the health care institution until the disease is noninfectious. *(p. 348)*

48. **(D)**   Bilirubin is light sensitive and will decrease in value if the blood for its collection is exposed to light. *(p. 148)*

49. (E) Bones are classified into four groups on the basis of their shapes: Long bones include leg bones and arm and hand bones. Short bones include wrist and ankle bones. Flat bones include several cranial bones, the ribs, and the shoulder blades. Irregular bones include some cranial bones and those of the vertebral column. *(p. 47)*

50. (E) Health care facilities in which blood collection usually occurs include health maintenance organizations (HMOs), multiphasic screening centers, community health centers, and medical group practices. *(pp. 7–8)*

51. (C) Normal human cells contain 46 chromosomes. *(p. 60)*

52. (D) The Joint Commission on Accreditation of Healthcare Organizations (JCAHO) uses a 10-step process for quality assessment of health care performance. *(p. 446)*

53. (A) *(p. 526)*

54. (C) The Autolet II Clinisafe device is for skin puncture collections. *(pp. 138, 146–147)*

55. (D) The term *stat* refers to an immediate or emergency condition. It indicates that a patient has a medical condition that is critical or likely to become critical. Stat blood collections should be collected and analyzed immediately. *(p. 189)*

56. (D) Edema is an abnormal accumulation of fluid in the intercellular spaces of the body. *(p. 207)*

57. (D) The digestive system functions, first, to break down food chemically and physically into nutrients that can be absorbed and used by body cells, and second, to eliminate the waste products of digestion. *(p. 56)*

58. (D) Personnel in the deoxyribonucleic acid (DNA) probe analysis section may test for genetic disorders, malignant disorders, infectious pathogens, or DNA fingerprinting in forensic medicine. *(p. 29)*

59. (B) The average depth of a skin puncture should be 2–3 mm to avoid hitting a bone. *(pp. 197-200)*

60. (A) A CVC is a central venous catheter. *(p. 258)*

61. (D) Teenagers are usually actively involved in anything concerning the body, embarrassed to show fear, and may act hostile to mask fear. *(p. 231)*

62. (B) Meninges are the protective membranes that cover the brain and spinal cord. *(p. 51)*

63. (A) Yellow-topped evacuated tubes containing sodium polyanethole sulfonate (SPS) may be used to collect specimens for blood culture determinations. *(p. 272)*

64. (C) A discussion of why a certain test was ordered or which tests were ordered is inappropriate. Requests for such information should be referred to the physician. *(pp. 480–481)*

65. (B) If a physician orders laboratory tests for diagnosis and the patient comes to the laboratory with a rolled-up sleeve, he/she is giving informed consent. *(p. 499)*

66. (D) The liver secretes bile. *(p. 57)*

67. (B) Physical medicine is the department for the diagnosis and treatment of disorders and disabilities of the neuromuscular system. *(p. 11)*

68. (D) To help minimize the incidence of dizziness, fainting, or other reactions to blood loss, blood donors are encouraged to eat within 4–6 hr. of donating blood. *(p. 290)*

69. (B) Insulin is secreted into the blood stream from the pancreas and leads to a decrease in blood glucose levels. *(p. 307)*

70. (A) Glomeruli are considered the filters of the kidney because they filter out water and solutes and reabsorb only the necessary amounts of these substances into the blood. Excess water and wastes are excreted as urine. *(p. 58)*

71. (D) When a skin puncture is performed on an infant or a child, hematology specimens are collected first to minimize platelet clumping. *(p. 238)*

72. (D) Two or three 20-mL disposable syringes and 10 mL of normal saline are needed to collect blood through central venous catheters (CVCs). *(p. 287)*

73. (D) Peritoneal fluid is collected from the sac around the heart. *(p. 330)*

74. (B) The endocrine system can best be evaluated by analyzing hormone levels. *(pp. 62–63)*

75. (A) Erythrocytes are red blood cells. *(p. 73)*

76. (A) Chromosome analysis requires whole blood collected in a green-topped blood collection tube. *(pp. 112, 122)*

77. (B) The needle should be inserted at a 15° angle to the skin. *(p. 173)*

78. (B) Personnel in the histology section are involved in the preparation and processing of tissue samples removed during surgery, autopsy, or other medical procedures. *(p. 28)*

79. (A) Physiology is the study of the functional components of the body. *(p. 38)*

80. (B) Thrombi are solid masses derived from blood constituents that reside in the blood vessels. *(p. 208)*

81. (D) Testing for trace metals involves the use of specially prepared trace metal evacuated blood collection tubes or special acid-washed plastic syringes. *(p. 285)*

82. (A) Na^+, K^+, Cl^-, and HCO^-_3 are usually referred to as *electrolytes*. *(p. 311)*

83. (A) *Escherichia coli* is a commonly identified pathogenic agent that causes nosocomial infections in the nursery unit. *(p. 346)*

84. (B) *(p. 529)*

85. (C) Before a patient's laboratory test results can legally be released, the patient must provide written consent. *(p. 505)*

86. **(A)** Customer satisfaction focuses on meeting the needs of those who are being served. *(p. 448)*

87. **(B)** Bar codes represent a series of light and dark bands of varying widths that depict alphanumeric symbols. *(pp. 419–420)*

88. **(C)** If an accident occurs, such as a needle stick, the health care provider should immediately cleanse the area with isopropyl alcohol and apply a Band-Aid. *(p. 383)*

89. **(B)** Hexachlorophene is an antiseptic for skin used frequently in surgery. *(p. 372)*

90. **(A)** A 24-hr. urine specimen is usually collected to test for hormones. *(p. 326)*

91. **(D)** Therapeutic phlebotomy is used in the treatment of some myeloproliferative diseases, such as polycythemia, or other conditions in which the removal of blood benefits the patient. *(p. 295)*

92. **(B)** Tylenol, or acetaminophen, use can lead to falsely increased values in liver function tests. *(pp. 214–215, 216)*

93. **(C)** Excessive massaging or milking of the puncture site can cause hemolysis and contamination of the blood specimen with tissue and intracellular fluids. *(p. 200)*

94. **(C)** All specimen labels should include the following information: patient's name and identification number, date and time of collection, and phlebotomist's initials. The patient's room number, bed assignment, or outpatient status is optional but useful information. *(p. 184)*

95. **(B)** The anticoagulant sodium heparin is found in a green-topped blood collection vacuum tube. *(p. 122)*

96. **(C)** Thrombocytes are platelets. *(p. 73)*

97. **(D)** The cell nucleus governs the functions of each cell. *(p. 41)*

98. (D) In the radiology department, ionizing radiation is used for treating disease, fluoroscopic and radiographic x-ray instrumentation are used for diagnosing disease, and radioactive isotopes are used for both diagnosing and treating disease. *(p. 12)*

99. (A) As CO_2 levels increase in the blood, the blood pH decreases (becomes more acidic). As the CO_2 level in the blood increases, chemoreceptors in the brain cause a faster and deeper rate of respiration (hyperventilation) in order to blow off excess CO_2 from the body. *(p. 55)*

100. (C) *(p. 529)*

Practice Test Questions 2

DIRECTIONS (Questions 1–20): Each of the questions or incomplete statements below is followed by suggested answers or completions. Select the **BEST** answer in each case.

AP   **1.** Anatomy is the study of

         A. the functional components of the body
         B. the biochemical makeup of the body
         C. the structural components of the body
         D. anabolic and catabolic mechanisms in the body

HCS   **2.** Specimens for clinical microbiological analysis must be handled with extreme care since they are a

         A. fire hazard
         B. radiation hazard
         C. biohazard
         D. chemical hazard

AP   **3.** What portion of human body weight is water?

       A. 90%
       B. 66%
       C. 50%
       D. 25%

CS   **4.** Plasma is blood

       A. that is highly oxygenated
       B. containing anticoagulant
       C. without anticoagulant
       D. rich in carbon monoxide

BCE   **5.** Specimens for blood gas analysis are collected in tubes with which of the following anticoagulants?

       A. EDTA
       B. Heparin
       C. Oxalate
       D. Citrate

BCE   **6.** Which of the following was introduced to help in the prevention of accidental needle sticks?

       A. Hemogard (Becton Dickinson VACUTAINER Systems, Franklin Lakes, NJ)
       B. Monoject Corvac tube (Sherwood Medical Monoject Division, St. Louis, MO)
       C. Microtainer (Becton Dickinson VACUTAINER Systems, Franklin Lakes, NJ)
       D. Safety-Gard Phlebotomy System (Becton Dickinson VACUTAINER Systems, Franklin Lakes, NJ)

VP **7.** Which of the following methods involves the use of a barrel and plunger to create a vacuum during venipuncture?

    A. Syringe method
    B. Tourniquet
    C. Capillary tube
    D. Evacuated tube method

SPP **8.** Which of the listed sequences is the **BEST** method for performing a finger stick?

    A. Squeeze the finger, decontaminate, puncture the skin
    B. Decontaminate, squeeze the finger, puncture the skin, collect the first drop
    C. Decontaminate, puncture the skin, wipe the first drop, collect the blood sample
    D. Apply a tourniquet, puncture the skin, wipe the first drop, collect the blood sample

CBC **9.** Another term for *fainting* is

    A. fomite
    B. syncope
    C. lymphostasis
    D. thrombus

PP **10.** EMLA is sometimes used for pediatric venipuncture procedures. EMLA is a

    A. local anesthetic applied with a small needle to the child's arm prior to venipuncture
    B. topical anesthetic applied to the child's arm prior to venipuncture
    C. topical lotion applied to the child's arm after venipuncture to stop bleeding at the venipuncture site
    D. topical lotion applied to the child's arm prior to venipuncture to avoid excessive bleeding at the site

ASC **11.** The health care worker's thumb should not be used for palpating arteries in the arterial puncture procedure because the thumb

    A. is usually dirty
    B. has less sensitivity than the other fingers
    C. has a pulse that may be confused with the patient's pulse
    D. has more neurons for touching, which interferes in the process of finding the patient's pulse

UBF **12.** Which of the following is obtained through a lumbar puncture?

    A. Pleural fluid
    B. Cerebrospinal fluid
    C. Synovial fluid
    D. Peritoneal fluid

IF **13.** Which of the following is **NOT** one of the links in the chain of infection?

    A. Susceptible host
    B. Poor isolation technique
    C. Source
    D. Mode of transmission

SFA **14.** Safe working conditions must be ensured by the employer and have been mandated by law under the

    A. Occupational Safety and Health Administration standards
    B. Institutional Safety and Health Act
    C. Health Care Facility Institutional Safety Act
    D. Occupational Safety and Hospital standards

TQM **15.** JCAHO is

    A. a proficiency testing company
    B. an accrediting agency for health care facilities
    C. an agency that administers certification examination
    D. a governmental agency that administers Medicare

ASC **16.** If the patient's bleeding time is longer than the normal limits, which of the following laboratory tests may be needed?

    A. Alkaline phosphatase
    B. Acid phosphatase
    C. Platelet count
    D. Blood urea nitrogen result

CPM **17.** The term *bedside manner* refers to

    A. a positive approach to the patient
    B. the phlebotomist's body position
    C. the patient's manners
    D. an analytic approach to bedside testing

LRI **18.** Examining witnesses before trial is referred to as

    A. discovery
    B. informed consent
    C. respondeat superior
    D. implied consent

AE **19.** From the following, select the most appropriate Spanish translation for the English phrase "I need to stick your finger."

    A. Necesito sacar sangre
    B. Le va a doler un poquito
    C. Necesito picarle su dedo
    D. Como se llama?

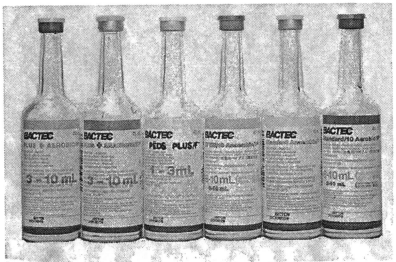

Figure 2-1 *(Courtesy of Becton Dickinson Microbiology Systems, Sparks, MD)*

BCE 20. The vials shown in Figure 2-1 are used in the collection of

A. immunohematology specimens
B. clinical chemistry specimens
C. clinical immunology specimens
D. microbiology specimens

DIRECTIONS (Questions 21–52): For each of the following questions or incomplete statements **ONE** or **MORE** of the numbered responses are correct. In each case, select

A. if only 1, 2, and 3 are correct
B. if only 1 and 3 are correct
C. if only 2 and 4 are correct
D. if only 4 is correct
E. if all are correct

HCS 21. In which of the following department(s) may personnel inject a patient with dyes and/or radioisotopes that can interfere in laboratory assays?

1. Physical therapy
2. Nuclear medicine
3. Occupational therapy
4. Radiology/medical imaging

AP 22. The nervous system is composed of which component(s)?

1. Brain
2. Spinal fluid
3. Spinal cord
4. Meninges

HCS 23. Which of the following terms appropriately classifies (classify) psychiatric hospitals?

1. Multiphasic screening centers
2. HMOs
3. Neighborhood health centers
4. Special-care hospitals

CS   **24.** All blood cells develop

      1. from undifferentiated stem cells
      2. every 180 days
      3. in the hematopoietic tissues
      4. as megakaryocytes before differentiating

BCE   **25.** The platelet function profile requires which of the following specimen types in a tube or tubes with what color(s) of top(s)?

      1. Whole blood (purple)
      2. Plasma (blue)
      3. Whole blood (blue)
      4. Serum (red)

AP   **26.** Which of the following pairs are opposite regions or planes of the body?

      1. Anterior/posterior
      2. Distal/proximal
      3. Lateral/medial
      4. Anterior/ventral

HCS   **27.** Which of the following laboratory personnel are listed **BELOW** the administrative technologist on the organizational chart of a typical clinical laboratory?

      1. Hematology supervisor
      2. Medical technologist
      3. Medical technician
      4. Phlebotomist

CS   **28.** RBCs are characterized by which of the following features?

     1. They measure about 7 μm diameter
     2. They have no nuclei when circulating in the peripheral blood
     3. They are biconcaved disks
     4. Their life span is about 120 days

BCE   **29.** Which of the following can be used in venipuncture procedure as a tourniquet?

     1. Velcro strap
     2. Seraket (Propper Manufacturing Co., Inc., Long Island City, NY)
     3. Latex strap
     4. Blood pressure cuff

SPP   **30.** Alcohol that has not dried on a skin puncture site can

     1. prevent a round drop of blood from forming
     2. cause hemolysis of blood cells
     3. cause erroneous results for some laboratory tests
     4. provide a more sterile puncture site

AP   **31.** Disorders of the skeletal system include

     1. arthritis and bursitis
     2. gout
     3. bacterial infections
     4. tumors

HCS   **32.** Sometimes, the health care worker must collect blood for analysis of serum lipids, which include

     1. creatinine
     2. triglycerides
     3. blood urea nitrogen (BUN)
     4. cholesterol

VP   **33.** Information on an inpatient's identification bracelet usually includes the

   1. patient's name
   2. patient's identification number
   3. patient's bed assignment
   4. physician's name

CBC   **34.** If a patient ate just before collection of a blood sample, what should the health care worker who is collecting the blood do?

   1. Collect the specimen
   2. Indicate what the patient ate
   3. Make a note that the patient was "nonfasting"
   4. Avoid collecting the specimen

PP   **35.** Which of the following pediatric conditions lead(s) to an elevated sensitivity to latex and latex allergy?

   1. Spina bifida
   2. Congenital urinary tract abnormalities
   3. Neurogenic bladder abnormality
   4. Multiple sclerosis

ASC   **36.** Which of the following can lead to errors in the collection of blood for blood cultures?

   1. Palpating the venipuncture site after the site has been prepared without first cleaning the gloved finger
   2. Injecting air into the anaerobic bottle
   3. Inoculating the anaerobic bottle last
   4. Wiping the iodine from the tops of the bottles with alcohol

HHB **37.** Which of the following instruments is (are) used in point-of-care (POC) glucose testing?

    1. Accu-Chek Easy (Boehringer Mannheim Corp., Mannheim, Federal Republic of Germany)
    2. AccuMeter (ChemTrak, Inc., Sunnyvale, CA)
    3. One Touch II Hospital (Life Scan, Mountain View, CA)
    4. i-STAT (i-STAT Corporation, Princeton, NJ)

UBF **38.** Which of the following might the health care worker need to transport to the laboratory for necessary analysis?

    1. Gastric secretions
    2. Peritoneal fluid
    3. Pleural fluid
    4. CSF

ASC **39.** Which of the following materials and/or supplies is (are) needed for the Surgicutt procedure?

    1. Blood pressure cuff
    2. Butterfly-type bandage
    3. Disposable gloves
    4. Vacuum blood collection tube with EDTA

TQM **40.** Customers in health care include

    1. patients or clients
    2. technologists, nurses
    3. physicians
    4. students

SDT   **41.** General guidelines for documenting information in a
medical record include

    1. accuracy
    2. completion
    3. objective reporting of facts
    4. covering up mistakes

CPM   **42.** An example of positive body language is

    1. staring at the ceiling and slouching in a chair
    2. smiling and making eye contact with a patient
    3. speaking in a monotone voice
    4. having erect posture

AE   **43.** *Degrees Fahrenheit* refers to

    1. a unit of temperature
    2. cubic millimeter
    3. °F
    4. degrees Celsius

HCS   **44.** A physician who usually has extensive education in the
study and diagnosis of diseases through the use of laboratory test results is sometimes referred to as

    1. a technical supervisor
    2. an administrative technologist
    3. a medical technologist
    4. a pathologist

CPM   **45.** The phlebotomist plays an active role in educating the patient about collecting specimens for which of the following tests?

       1. Glucose tolerance tests
       2. Urine cultures
       3. 24-hr. urine samples
       4. Routine hematology tests

CBC   **46.** The term *fasting* usually means abstaining from

       1. water
       2. everything
       3. smoking
       4. food and drinks other than water

CS   **47.** The blood vessels that carry oxygenated blood away from the heart are

       1. capillaries
       2. venules
       3. veins
       4. arteries

ASC   **48.** Before blood donation, the phlebotomist must always check the blood donor's

       1. blood glucose value or urine glucose value
       2. hematocrit or hemoglobin value
       3. WBC count
       4. temperature

IC 　　**49.** Which of the following can make a patient a potential host for a nosocomial infection?

    1. Chemotherapy
    2. Cancer
    3. Antibiotics
    4. Acquired immunodeficiency syndrome (AIDS)

IC 　　**50.** Babies whose mothers have which of the following conditions must be isolated from other infants?

    1. Burns
    2. Cancer
    3. Kidney failure and are in a dialysis unit
    4. Genital herpes

BCE 　　**51.** Lithium heparin is a suitable anticoagulant for which of the following studies?

    1. Glucose level
    2. BUN level
    3. Creatinine level
    4. Ionized calcium level

SPP 　　**52.** The finger-stick procedure involves which of the following steps?

    1. The patient's finger should be held firmly, with the phlebotomist's thumb away from the puncture site
    2. The puncture should be performed in one sharp, continuous movement
    3. The puncture should be perpendicular to the skin
    4. The puncture should be across the fingerprint

DIRECTIONS (Questions 53–100): Each of the questions or incomplete statements below is followed by suggested answers or completions. Select the **BEST** answer in each case.

SFA   **53.** If a chemical is spilled onto a health care worker, he/she should first

    A. rub vigorously with a disinfectant
    B. wait and see if it starts to burn the skin
    C. rinse the area with a neutral chemical
    D. rinse the area with water

CBC   **54.** *Supine* refers to

    A. sitting
    B. standing
    C. lying
    D. hemolysis

AP   **55.** The pituitary gland is often referred to as which of the following?

    A. Respiratory control gland
    B. Master gland
    C. Lymph tissue
    D. Germ cells

AE   **56.** The phrase "It will hurt a little" in Spanish is

    A. Necesito sacar sangre
    B. Le va a doler un poquito
    C. Necesito picarle su dedo
    D. Como se llama?

UBF   **57.** Fluid composed of products formed in various male reproductive organs is referred to as

     A. pleural fluid
     B. seminal fluid
     C. synovial fluid
     D. cerebrospinal fluid

ASC   **58.** The Isostat system (Wampole Laboratories, Cranbury, NJ) is a

     A. special arterial blood gas syringe
     B. special blood culture tube system
     C. bleeding-time system
     D. peripheral catheter system

LRI   **59.** When specimens are collected for toxicological studies involving drug abuse testing, these specimens are referred to as

     A. FDA specimens
     B. forensic specimens
     C. EPA specimens
     D. CDC specimens

AP   **60.** The skeletal system provides which of the body's functions?

     A. Elimination of wastes
     B. Hormone secretion and equilibrium maintenance
     C. Facilitates respiration by expansion/contraction of rib cage
     D. Blood cell formation, calcium storage, leverage, and movement

HCS   **61.** A health care worker who collects blood in a health care facility that has only elderly patients works in which of the following?

       A. Obstetrics facility
       B. Geriatrics facility
       C. Pediatrics facility
       D. Neonatal facility

VP   **62.** How many seconds prior to the venipuncture should the alcohol be allowed to dry?

       A. 0–5
       B. 5–10
       C. 10–15
       D. 30–60

IC   **63.** Which of the following illnesses can result in enteric isolation?

       A. Mumps
       B. Measles
       C. Rubella
       D. Amebic dysentery

PP   **64.** When collecting blood from a heparin lock on a child, the phlebotomist must check the patency of the line by

       A. disinfecting the catheter cap with alcohol or povidone-iodine solution
       B. flushing with a small amount of normal saline
       C. injecting slowly the heparinized flush solution
       D. flushing with a small amount of glucose solution

SDT **65.** The Hazard Communication Standard relates to

    A. procedures and documentation regarding hazardous substances
    B. quality control procedures and quality assurance standards
    C. policies about clinical competency
    D. instrument and maintenance records for equipment

AP **66.** Diffusion between air and blood takes place in which anatomical area?

    A. Glomeruli
    B. Cardiac muscle
    C. Alveolar sacs
    D. Nasal passages

CS **67.** Leukocytes function primarily to

    A. transport oxygen
    B. provide host cells
    C. promote clotting
    D. defend against infections

SPP **68.** What should the phlebotomist do with the first drop of blood when a finger stick is performed?

    A. Use it for chemistry testing
    B. Make a blood smear or slide
    C. Wipe it off with gauze
    D. Use it for hematology testing

VP   **69.** Which of the following methods causes "pooling" of blood in veins?

    A. Syringe method
    B. Tourniquet application
    C. Capillary tube
    D. Evacuated tube method

HCS   **70.** A health care worker has to collect blood from patients in the nephrology department, the department for diagnosis and treatment of problems related to the

    A. lungs
    B. heart
    C. kidneys
    D. nervous system

AP   **71.** TSH, T_3, and T_4 are diagnostic tests useful in detecting abnormalities for which of the following?

    A. Blood clotting
    B. Thyroid function
    C. Diabetes
    D. None of the above

UBF   **72.** Amniotic fluid can be found

    A. around the lungs
    B. surrounding the heart
    C. around the fetus in the uterus
    D. surrounding the liver, the pancreas, and other parts of the gastrointestinal area

IC 73. A nosocomial infection occurs when

    A. a source is detected
    B. the chain of infection is complete
    C. a means of transmission is maintained by disinfectants
    D. a susceptible host remains stable

CPM 74. A phlebotomist can make a positive or negative impression on a patient within

    A. 30 min.
    B. 5 min.
    C. 60 sec.
    D. 30 sec.

HHB 75. The blood analyte(s) that is (are) tested by the HemoCue analyzers is (are)

    A. cholesterol
    B. glucose and hemoglobin
    C. PT and APTT
    D. hemoglobin and hematocrit

ASC 76. Which of the following procedures helps reduce potential scarring from the Surgicutt bleeding-time test?

    A. Apply a butterfly-type bandage to the incision site
    B. Provide a small stitch to the incision site
    C. Apply gauze and tape to the incision site
    D. Apply a small piece of moleskin to the incision site

CBC **77.** Small red spots that appear on a patient's skin and indicate that minute amounts of blood have escaped into skin epithelium are

A. hemoconcentration
B. hemolysis
C. petechiae
D. thrombi

AE **78.** Which of the following is the correct phrase in Spanish for "What is your name?"

A. Ya tomo el desayuno?
B. Como esta usted?
C. Necesito picarle su dedo
D. Como se llama?

LRI **79.** Failure to act or perform duties according to standards of the profession is

A. battery
B. negligence
C. criminal action
D. slander

BCE **80.** Which of the following is a serum separation tube?

A. Heparinized Natelson tube
B. Seraket
C. Winged infusion set
D. Monoject Corvac tube

SDT **81.** Using an airtight container and ice water to transport an arterial specimen for blood gas analysis is useful because

    A. it decreases the loss of gases from the specimen
    B. it promotes coagulation and fibrinolysis
    C. it aids in the instrumentation phase of the testing process
    D. it increases the oxygen content in the specimen

HCS **82.** Rheumatology can best be described as a department for

    A. diagnosis and treatment of rheumatic fever
    B. correction of the loss or deformity of tissues, including skin
    C. diagnosis and treatment of diseases of the anus and rectum
    D. diagnosis and treatment of joint and tissue diseases, including arthritis

IC **83.** Which of the following is not a factor that links the susceptible host to the source in the chain of infection?

    A. Chemotherapy
    B. Immunosuppression
    C. Radiation therapy
    D. Good nutrition

SFA **84.** Chemicals defined as "explosive flammables" must be stored

    A. in a cabinet under the sink
    B. in small carrying containers
    C. on a high shelf away from light and heat
    D. in an explosion-proof or a fireproof room or cabinet

AP   **85.** Respiratory acidosis occurs in which of the following cases?

       A. When the pH of the blood falls below 7.35
       B. When the respiratory system is not able to eliminate adequate amounts of carbon dioxide
       C. Conditions such as a collapsed lung or blockage of respiratory passages
       D. All of the above

VP   **86.** During the venipuncture procedure, after the needle is inserted and blood begins to flow, what should the phlebotomist do next?

       A. Release the tourniquet
       B. Withdraw the needle
       C. Release the luer
       D. Adjust the hub of the needle

AP   **87.** Disorders of the lymphatic system include which of the following?

       A. Lymphoma
       B. Hodgkin's disease
       C. Immune disorders
       D. All of the above

PP   **88.** The angle of the needle for scalp vein venipuncture of an infant should be

       A. 15°
       B. 30°
       C. 60°
       D. 90°

ASC   **89.** Which of the following is used to help in the diagnosis of diabetes mellitus?

    A. GTT
    B. ABG
    C. TDM
    D. CVC

AP   **90.** Disorders of the nervous system include which of the following conditions?

    A. Encephalitis
    B. Meningitis and Parkinson's disease
    C. Amyotrophic lateral sclerosis
    D. All of the above

HCS   **91.** Cerebrospinal fluid (CSF), biopsy specimens, and gastric secretions are analyzed in which department?

    A. Radiation therapy
    B. Radiology/medical imaging
    C. Physical medicine
    D. Clinical laboratory

BCE   **92.** Which of the following is (are) frequently used for the microcollection of specimens for blood gas analysis?

    A. Unopette
    B. Heparinized Natelson tubes (100–250 uL)
    C. Microtainer
    D. Autolet Lite Clinisafe

AE   **93.** One inch equals

    A. 1 cm
    B. 1 mm
    C. 5.45 cm
    D. 2.54 cm

LRI   **94.** In legal cases, "what a reasonably prudent person would do under similar circumstances" refers to

    A. discovery
    B. standard of care
    C. informed consent
    D. standard policies and procedures

BCE   **95.** Which of the following tests requires plasma collected in a purple-topped vacuum tube and transported in ice water?

    A. Bleeding-time test
    B. Leukocyte alkaline phosphatase level
    C. Erythrocyte fragility test
    D. Renin activity test

IC   **96.** Which of the following is a commonly identified pathogenic microorganism that causes skin nosocomial infections?

    A. *Candida albicans*
    B. *Haemophilus vaginalis*
    C. *Shigella sp.*
    D. *Moraxella lacunata*

CPM   **97.** The Patient's Bill of Rights

    A. serves as a pledge of appropriate behavior for physicians
    B. describes the rights of patients in a health care environment
    C. describes ethical conduct for physicians
    D. describes the principle of informed consent

SPP   **98.** The best angle for spreading a blood smear by using two glass slides is

     A. 15°
     B. 30°
     C. 45°
     D. 90°

CS   **99.** Erythrocytes function primarily to

     A. transport oxygen
     B. provide host cells
     C. promote clotting
     D. defend against infections

HCS   **100.** Which of the following is an instrument usually found in the encephalography department?

     A. ECK
     B. EKG
     C. EEG
     D. EGK

Practice Test Questions 2

Answers and Discussion

Page numbers refer to Garza D, Becan-McBride K: *Phlebotomy Handbook, 4th ed.* Stamford, CT, Appleton & Lange, 1996.

1. **(C)**   Anatomy is the study of structural components of the body. *(p. 38)*

2. **(C)**   Specimens for microbiological analysis may be highly infectious and thus are considered biohazardous. *(p. 27)*

3. **(B)**   Approximately 66% of the human body is composed of water. *(p. 58)*

4. **(B)**   Plasma is blood that contains an anticoagulant and therefore does not form a clot. *(p. 78)*

5. **(B)**   Heparinized tubes are used to collect specimens for blood gas analysis. *(pp. 139–140)*

6. **(D)**   The Safety-Gard Phlebotomy System is a safety device that helps prevent accidental needle sticks. *(p. 105)*

7. **(A)**   The syringe method uses a barrel and plunger to create a vacuum during venipuncture. *(p. 174)*

8. **(C)** The most appropriate sequence for a skin puncture is to decontaminate, puncture the skin, wipe the first drop, then collect the blood sample. *(p. 196)*

9. **(B)** Another term for *fainting* is *syncope*. *(p. 204)*

10. **(B)** EMLA is a topical anesthetic applied to the child's arm prior to venipuncture. *(p. 235)*

11. **(C)** The health care provider's thumb should not be used for palpating arteries in the arterial puncture procedure because the thumb has a pulse that may be confused with the patient's pulse. *(p. 264)*

12. **(B)** Cerebrospinal fluid (CSF) is obtained through a spinal tap or lumbar puncture. *(p. 328)*

13. **(B)** The chain of infection comprises (1) susceptible host, (2) source, and (3) mode of transmission. *(p. 347)*

14. **(A)** Safe working conditions must be ensured by the employer and have been mandated by law under the Occupational Safety and Health Administration (OSHA) standards. *(p. 380)*

15. **(B)** JCAHO is the Joint Commission on Accreditation of Healthcare Organizations, a nonprofit agency that accredits health care facilities. *(p. 402)*

16. **(C)** A prolonged bleeding time may necessitate a platelet count. *(p. 269)*

17. **(A)** Bedside manner is established by being prepared and well equipped and by having a professional attitude, a pleasant facial expression, and a neat appearance. *(p. 466)*

18. **(A)** Discovery refers to examining witnesses before the trial to learn more about the legal case involved. *(p. 502)*

19. **(C)** *(p. 526)*

20. (D) The vials shown in Figure 2-1 are BACTEC culture vials for microbiology specimens (Becton Dickinson Microbiology Systems, Sparks, MD). *(p. 123)*

21. (C) Radiology/medical imaging studies sometimes require that the patient be injected with dye. Radioisotopes are injected intravenously into patients in the nuclear medicine department for diagnostic and treatment purposes. *(pp. 12–13)*

22. (E) The brain, spinal cord and fluid, and meninges are all functional components of the nervous system. *(p. 51)*

23. (D) Psychiatric hospitals are special-care hospitals, since they treat only a few types of illnesses. *(p. 9)*

24. (B) All blood cells develop from undifferentiated stem cells in the hematopoietic (blood-forming) tissues, such as the bone marrow. *(p. 73)*

25. (B) For the platelet function profile, whole blood collected in a purple-topped vacuum tube and whole blood collected in a blue-topped vacuum tube are needed. *(p. 118)*

26. (A) Opposite regions or planes of the body are anterior/posterior, distal/proximal, and lateral/medial. *(p. 40)*

27. (E) The administrative technologist oversees the activities of the hematology supervisor, medical technologist, medical technician, and phlebotomist. Thus, they are all listed below the administrative technologist on the organizational chart. *(p. 19)*

28. (E) RBCs measure about 7 μm in diameter, have no nuclei when circulating in the peripheral blood, are biconcaved disks, and have a life span of about 120 days. *(pp. 74–75)*

29. (E) Tourniquets that are used in venipuncture include the Velcro strap, the Seraket, the latex strap, and the blood pressure cuff. *(p. 134)*

30. (A) Alcohol that has not dried on a skin puncture site can prevent a round drop of blood from forming, cause hemolysis of blood cells, and cause erroneous results for some laboratory tests such as glucose determinations. *(p. 197)*

31. **(E)** Disorders of the skeletal system include inflammatory conditions such as arthritis and bursitis; gout; bacterial infections such as osteomyelitis; porous bone conditions such as osteoporosis; developmental conditions such as gigantism, dwarfism, and rickets; and bone marrow diseases. *(p. 48)*

32. **(C)** Serum lipids are the triglycerides and cholesterol; assays of serum lipids are usually performed in the clinical chemistry area. *(p. 22)*

33. **(E)** Information on the patient's identification bracelet may include the patient's name, identification number, bed assignment, birth date, and room number, and the physician's name. *(pp. 157, 158)*

34. **(B)** If a patient ate just before blood collection, the blood specimen(s) should be collected and a note should be made that the patient was "nonfasting." *(p. 210)*

35. **(A)** Children with spina bifida and those with congenital urinary tract abnormalities or neurogenic bladders are particularly sensitive to latex. *(p. 237)*

36. **(A)** The following can lead to errors in the collection of blood for blood cultures: (1) palpating the venipuncture site after the site has been prepared without first cleaning the gloved finger, (2) injecting air into the anaerobic bottle, and (3) inoculating the anaerobic bottle last. *(p. 275)*

37. **(B)** The Accu-Chek Easy and One Touch II Hospital are two POC glucose testing analyzers. *(p. 307)*

38. **(E)** The health care worker may become involved in transporting gastric secretions, peritoneal fluid, pleural fluid, and/or CSF to the laboratory. *(pp. 328, 332–333)*

39. **(A)** A blood pressure cuff (sphygmomanometer), a butterfly-type bandage, and disposable gloves are needed for the Surgicutt procedure. *(p. 267)*

40. **(E)** Customers in health care include patients or clients, technologists, nurses, physicians, and students. *(pp. 448, 451)*

41. **(A)** Documenting information in a medical record requires accuracy, completion, and objectivity. Records should *never* be erased or falsified to cover mistakes. *(p. 404)*

42. **(C)** Examples of positive body language include smiling, eye contact, erect posture, and professional appearance. *(p. 472)*

43. **(B)** *(p. 527)*

44. **(D)** The pathologist is a physician who has extensive education in pathology (the study and diagnosis of diseases through the use of laboratory test results). *(p. 17)*

45. **(A)** The phlebotomist plays an active role in patient education about glucose tolerance tests, urine cultures, and 24-hr. urine samples. *(p. 468)*

46. **(D)** *Fasting* usually means abstaining from food and drinks other than water. *(p. 210)*

47. **(D)** Blood vessels that carry blood away from the heart are arteries, and blood vessels that carry blood to the heart are veins. *(pp. 82–83)*

48. **(C)** The blood bank phlebotomist must check the blood donor's temperature and hematocrit or hemoglobin value before the blood donation. *(p. 291)*

49. **(E)** Chemotherapy, cancer, antibiotics, and AIDS can all change the status of the human body and make it a potential host for a nosocomial infection. *(p. 351)*

50. **(D)** Babies whose mothers have genital herpes must be isolated from other infants. *(p. 364)*

51. **(A)** Lithium heparin tubes may be used for glucose, BUN, creatinine, and electrolyte specimens. The anticoagulant is not suitable for specimens requiring the measurement of ionized calcium levels. *(p. 122)*

52. (E) During the finger-stick procedure, the patient's finger should be held firmly, with the phlebotomist's thumb away from the puncture site; the puncture should be performed in one sharp, continuous movement; the puncture should be perpendicular to the skin; and the puncture should be across the fingerprint. *(p. 197)*

53. (D) The victim of a chemical accident must immediately rinse the affected area with water for at least 15 min. after removing contaminated clothing. *(p. 390)*

54. (C) *Supine* refers to the lying position. *(p. 212)*

55. (B) The pituitary is often referred to as the master gland because it controls and regulates many functions of the body through hormone production. *(p. 62)*

56. (B) *(p. 526)*

57. (B) Seminal fluid is composed of products formed in various male reproductive organs. *(p. 329)*

58. (B) The Isostat system is a special blood culture tube system. *(p. 275)*

59. (B) When specimens are collected for toxicological studies involving drug abuse testing, these specimens are referred to as *forensic specimens*. *(p. 500)*

60. (D) The skeletal system provides bodily support and allows for leverage and movement. It also protects tissues, and plays a role in hematopoiesis (blood cell formation) in the bone marrow and in mineral storage. *(p. 47)*

61. (B) Geriatrics refers to the diagnosis and treatment of the elderly population. *(p. 11)*

62. (D) Alcohol should be allowed to dry for 30 to 60 sec. or should be wiped off with sterile gauze or cotton after the site is prepared. If not dry, the alcohol will cause the puncture site to sting and/or may interfere with test results such as blood alcohol levels. *(p. 171)*

63. (D) Amebic dysentery and other parasitic infections can result in enteric isolation. *(p. 356)*

64. (B) When collecting blood from a heparin lock on a child, the phlebotomist must check the patency of the line by flushing with a small amount of normal saline. *(p. 251)*

65. (A) The Hazard Communication Standard enacted in 1986 requires that employers maintain documentation related to any hazardous substances. Employers must have a written communication program and must provide training for employees, documentation about hazardous substances, MSDS, biohazard labels, and ways to react to accidents. *(p. 411)*

66. (C) Oxygen and carbon dioxide exchange actually takes place in the alveolar sacs within the bronchi. Alveoli are grapelike sacs where air diffusion occurs into the blood. *(p. 54)*

67. (D) The primary function of leukocytes is to provide a defense against pathogenic organisms. *(p. 77)*

68. (C) The first drop of blood from a finger stick should be wiped off with gauze. *(p. 200)*

69. (B) A tourniquet causes pooling of blood in veins. Such pooling makes blood collection easier during a venipuncture procedure. *(p. 170)*

70. (C) The nephrology department is concerned with the diagnosis and treatment of kidney diseases. *(p. 12)*

71. (B) Thyroid function abnormalities can be detected by the following diagnostic tests: thyroid stimulating hormone (TSH), triiodothyronine (T_3), and thyroxine (T_4). *(p. 63)*

72. (C) Amniotic fluid surrounds the fetus in the uterus. *(p. 329)*

73. (B) Nosocomial infections occur when the chain of infection is complete. The three components that make up the chain are source, mode of transmission, and susceptible host. *(p. 347)*

74. (D) The first 30 sec. after the phlebotomist enters the patient's room determines how that patient perceives the phlebotomist and the quality of the care that he/she is receiving. *(p. 466)*

75. (B) Blood glucose and hemoglobin are the analyzers tested by the HemoCue analyzers. *(p. 307)*

76. (A) Applying a butterfly-type bandage to the incision area for a 24-hr. period can reduce the scarring that may result from a Surgicutt bleeding-time test. *(p. 267)*

77. (C) Petechiae are small red spots that appear on the skin and indicate that minute amounts of blood have escaped into skin epithelium. *(p. 206)*

78. (D) *(p. 526)*

79. (B) Failure to act or perform duties according to standards of the profession is negligence. *(p. 495)*

80. (D) The Monoject Corvac tube is a serum separation tube. *(p. 123)*

81. (A) Using an airtight container and ice water to transport an arterial specimen for blood gas analysis decreases the loss of gases (oxygen and carbon dioxide) from the specimen. *(p. 427)*

82. (D) Rheumatology is the department concerned with the diagnosis and treatment of joint and tissue diseases, including arthritis. *(p. 11)*

83. (D) Good nutrition interrupts the chain of nosocomial infection between the susceptible host and the source. *(p. 351)*

84. (D) Explosive flammables must be stored in an explosion-proof or fireproof room or cabinet. *(p. 390)*

85. (D) Respiratory acidosis occurs during respiratory failure when the pH of the blood falls below 7.35, when the respiratory system is not able to eliminate adequate amounts of carbon dioxide, as in conditions such as collapsed lung or blockage of respiratory passages. *(p. 59)*

86. (A) After the needle is inserted and blood begins to flow, the tourniquet should be released and the patient may open his/her fist. *(pp. 173–174)*

87. (D) Disorders involving the lymphatic system are tumors (such as lymphoma) and Hodgkin's disease, immune disorders, and infectious processes. *(p. 65)*

88. (A) Position the needle at a 15° angle over the vein in the direction of the blood flow for scalp vein venipuncture of an infant. *(p. 250)*

89. (A) The glucose tolerance test (GTT) is frequently used to help in the diagnosis of diabetes mellitus. *(p. 276)*

90. (D) Disorders of the nervous system include encephalitis, meningitis, tetanus, herpes, and poliomyelitis, and conditions such as amyotrophic lateral sclerosis, multiple sclerosis, Parkinson's disease, cerebral palsy, tumors, epilepsy, hydrocephaly, neuralgia, and headaches. *(pp. 51–52)*

91. (D) The clinical laboratory department analyzes various body fluids and tissues, including cerebrospinal fluid (CSF), biopsy specimens, and gastric secretions. *(p. 16)*

92. (B) Heparinized Natelson tubes (100–250 uL) are frequently used for the microcollection of specimens for blood gas analysis. *(pp. 139–140)*

93. (D) *(p. 529)*

94. (B) In legal cases, the standard of care is determined by what a reasonably prudent person would do under similar circumstances. *(p. 498)*

95. (D) The renin activity assay requires plasma collected in a purple-topped vacuum tube and transported in ice water. *(p. 119)*

96. (A) *Candida albicans* is a commonly identified pathogenic agent that causes skin nosocomial infections. *(p. 347)*

97. (B)   The Patient's Bill of Rights describes the rights of patients in a health care environment. Key elements include patients' rights to respectful, considerate care; accurate information; informed consent; refusal of treatment; privacy; confidentiality; information about who his/her provider is; information about procedures for research; and billing information. *(p. 480)*

98. (B)   The best angle for spreading a blood smear by using two glass slides is 30°. *(p. 199)*

99. (A)   The primary function of erythrocytes is to transport oxygen (O_2). *(p. 74)*

100. (C)   The encephalography department uses the electroencephalograph (EEG), which records brain waves. *(p. 15)*

Practice Test Questions 3

DIRECTIONS (Questions 1–25): For each of the following questions or incomplete statements, **ONE** or **MORE** of the numbered responses are correct. In each case, select

    A. if only 1, 2, and 3 are correct
    B. if only 1 and 3 are correct
    C. if only 2 and 4 are correct
    D. if only 4 is correct
    E. if all are correct

AE   **1.** The symbol L refers to

    1. less than
    2. likely to be
    3. Likert scale
    4. liter

LRI   **2.** Confidential patient information and materials include

    1. a patient's verbal statements
    2. laboratory test results
    3. conversations between the physician and the patient
    4. employee drug testing report

CPM   **3.** For a 24-hr. urine collection, the patient should be advised to

      1. save the first morning specimen
      2. void at 7:00 AM and discard the urine
      3. collect urine for 12 hr.
      4. collect all urine for the next 24 hr. in the container provided

TQM   **4.** The speed of a centrifuge can be checked by a tachometer, which indicates

      1. RPM
      2. circumference of the centrifuge
      3. revolutions per minute
      4. the g value

SDT   **5.** PROs use medical records to

      1. evaluate the quality of care
      2. document medical stability
      3. evaluate the medical necessity of tests
      4. determine occurrence of avoidable tests

AP   **6.** The integumentary system consists of

      1. skin and hair
      2. sweat and oil glands
      3. teeth
      4. fingernails

AP   **7.** Functions of the skin include which of the following?

      1. Prevents water loss
      2. Secretes oils
      3. Produces perspiration
      4. Regulates hormone excretion

LRI   **8.** Key points in **ALL** negligence cases include

         1. duty and breach of duty
         2. invasion of privacy
         3. proximate causation and damages
         4. informed consent

ASC   **9.** Which of the following statements is (are) true regarding the Isostat system?

         1. It is a special blood culture tube system
         2. It has lysing and anticoagulating agents
         3. It has reagents in the tube that inactivate HIV
         4. It has containment adapters that help protect against breakage during centrifugation

VP   **10.** All requisitions for laboratory tests should contain which of the following information?

         1. Patient's full name and identification number
         2. Patient's date of birth
         3. Dates and types of tests to be performed
         4. Physician's name

BCE   **11.** Which of the following is (are) blood test(s) for syphilis?

         1. RPR
         2. TSH
         3. VDRL
         4. ALT

CS   **12.** The upper chambers of the heart are which of the following?

         1. Right atrium
         2. Right ventricle
         3. Left atrium
         4. Left ventricle

AP   **13.** Melanin

    1. is a pigment that provides skin color
    2. is a covering for the brain and spinal cord
    3. protects tissues from absorbing ultraviolet rays
    4. acts as a heat insulator

HCS   **14.** If a health care worker has a request to collect blood from a patient for serum electrolyte analysis, the assays performed in clinical chemistry will include

    1. sodium
    2. potassium
    3. chloride
    4. carbon monoxide

AE   **15.** The symbol $\geq$ means

    1. is negative
    2. is less than or equal to
    3. is positive
    4. is greater than or equal to

SDT   **16.** Disclosure of confidential information can result in

    1. a breach of the patient's rights
    2. a patient's improved understanding of his/her medical condition
    3. an invasion of the patient's privacy
    4. safe handling of patient test results

SFA   **17.** The ABC fire extinguisher can be used for

    1. electrical fires
    2. solvent fires
    3. paper fires
    4. plastic material fires

IC   **18.** Good technique in hand washing for the prevention of disease transmission in hospitals involves

     1. warm running water
     2. soap
     3. friction
     4. hand lotion or oil

UBF   **19.** The presence of which of the following constituents is tested for during chemical analysis in a routine urinalysis?

     1. Protein
     2. Bilirubin
     3. Hemoglobin
     4. Crystals

HHB   **20.** Which of the following terms is (are) synonymous with *POC testing*?

     1. On-site testing
     2. Alternate-site testing
     3. Near-patient testing
     4. Patient-focused testing

ASC   **21.** Blood glucose levels are measured for patients undergoing the

     1. glucagon tolerance test
     2. epinephrine tolerance test
     3. lactose tolerance test
     4. D-xylose tolerance test

AP   **22.** Which of the following body systems has (have) the functions of communication, control, and integration?

     1. Endocrine
     2. Reproductive
     3. Nervous
     4. Skeletal

HCS   **23.** When a *C&S* test is requested in the clinical microbiology department, this term refers to

     1. culturing and identifying bacterial pathogens and testing for inhibition of their growth by an antibiotic
     2. chemical testing and selectivity testing
     3. culture and sensitivity testing
     4. microscopic examination to identify crystals and casts

CS   **24.** Chambers of the heart include which of the following?

     1. Right and left atria
     2. Right ventricle
     3. Left ventricle
     4. Aortic chamber

PP   **25.** Which of the following blood collection items is (are) needed for a scalp vein venipuncture?

     1. 23- or 25-gauge winged infusion set
     2. Large, flat rubber band
     3. Disposable razor
     4. 23 × 3/4 in. transparent hub needle

DIRECTIONS (Questions 26–39): Each of the questions or incomplete statements below is followed by suggested answers or completions. Select the **BEST** answer in each case.

VP **26.** Which of the following methods requires a double-pointed needle?

    A. Syringe method
    B. Tourniquet
    C. Capillary tube
    D. Evacuated tube method

BCE **27.** Which of the following anticoagulants is found in a royal-blue-topped blood collection vacuum tube?

    A. EDTA
    B. No anticoagulant
    C. Sodium citrate
    D. Ammonium heparin

AE **28.** How is the phrase, "Have you had breakfast?" stated in Spanish?

    A. Ya tomo el desayuno?
    B. Entiende usted?
    C. Como se llama?
    D. Quien es us doctor?

LRI **29.** Which of the following agencies evaluates the safety, clinical efficacy, and medical efficacy of the equipment and supplies used in blood collection?

    A. FDA
    B. EPA
    C. OSHA
    D. CDC

TQM   **30.** CQI refers to the improvement of health care structures, processes, and outcomes, and client satisfaction. QC procedures refer to monitoring only

    A. structure
    B. process
    C. outcome
    D. client satisfaction

AP   **31.** Respiration in the average person is characterized by which of the following?

    A. Allows for the exchange of gases between blood and air
    B. Inhaling and exhaling occurs about 15 times per minute
    C. It occurs approximately 20,000 times per day
    D. All of the above

CS   **32.** Systole is

    A. contraction of the heart
    B. relaxation of the heart
    C. blood tension
    D. a heart murmur

CBC   **33.** Falsely decreased laboratory test results for a blood analyte can be

    A. mistakenly interpreted as normal when the blood analyte is truly in the subnormal range
    B. caused by increasing the color produced in the laboratory test
    C. mistakenly interpreted as normal or subnormal if the blood analyte is truly in an elevated range or normal range, respectively
    D. both a and b

SPP   **34.** Warming a site for skin puncture

        A. increases blood pressure
        B. increases blood flow to the site
        C. relaxes the patient
        D. eliminates the need for a tourniquet

SDT   **35.** The most efficient and accurate method of making specimen labels is by

        A. using physicians' orders from a Kardox
        B. using a hospital computer system
        C. manually labeling specimens at the bedside
        D. using the log sheets to determine which laboratory tests are ordered

BCE   **36.** Which of the following is a commonly used intravenous device that is sometimes used in the collection of blood from patients who are difficult to stick by conventional methods?

        A. Heparinized Natelson tube
        B. Unopette
        C. Butterfly needle
        D. Microtainer

HCS   **37.** The largest group of nongovernmental hospitals is referred to as

        A. community hospitals
        B. psychiatric hospitals
        C. Veterans Administration hospitals
        D. health maintenance hospitals

HCS   **38.** Which of the following best describes the department of electrocardiography?

    A. It is composed of clinical pathology and anatomic pathology
    B. It records the electric current produced by the contractions of the heart muscle
    C. It records the brain waves of the patient
    D. It uses radioactive material in the diagnosis and treatment of patients and in the study of the disease process

AP   **39.** Sensory neurons are defined by which of the following characteristics?

    A. Transmit nerve impulses from the spinal cord or brain to the muscles
    B. Nerve impulses from muscle tissues go to the brain or spinal cord
    C. Cause emotional problems
    D. None of the above

DIRECTIONS (Questions 40–56): For each of the following questions or incomplete statements **ONE** or **MORE** of the numbered responses are correct. In each case, select

    A. if only 1, 2, and 3 are correct
    B. if only 1 and 3 are correct
    C. if only 2 and 4 are correct
    D. if only 4 is correct
    E. if all are correct

SDT   **40.** Assays that may require chilled specimens include

    1. gastrin, ammonia, and lactic acid determinations
    2. renin, catecholamine, and parathyroid hormone determinations
    3. PT, PTT, and glucagon determinations
    4. blood gas analysis

BCE   **41.** Which of the following anticoagulant(s) is (are) used frequently in coagulation blood studies?

1. Citrate-phosphate-dextrose (CPD)
2. Sodium oxalate
3. Acid-citrate-dextrose
4. Sodium citrate

CS   **42.** Which of the following statements describe(s) plasma?

1. It contains clotted blood
2. It is obtained by mixing blood with an anticoagulant
3. It is normally bright yellow to orange
4. It is the fluid portion of unclotted blood

AP   **43.** The kidney's main function is to regulate which of the following in the body?

1. The amount of water
2. Electrolytes (sodium, potassium, chloride)
3. Nitrogenous waste products (urea)
4. Hemoglobin concentration

HCS   **44.** The clinical laboratory department is composed of which of the following areas?

1. Clinical pharmacy
2. Clinical pathology
3. Clinical encephalography
4. Anatomic pathology

AE   **45.** The symbol K refers to

1. Kelvin
2. kilograms
3. a unit of temperature
4. kilo-

TQM   **46.** Examples of outcome assessments for quality improvement involve evaluating

    1. recovery rates
    2. cure rates
    3. nosocomial infection rates
    4. return-to-normal-function rates

CPM   **47.** Positive body language includes

    1. maintaining erect posture
    2. smiling
    3. making eye contact
    4. bleeding-time tests

SFA   **48.** Which of the following organizations regulate(s) the disposal of wastes?

    1. EPA
    2. NCCLS
    3. OSHA
    4. NFPA

IC   **49.** Vectors in transmitting infectious diseases include

    1. age
    2. mosquitoes
    3. rabies
    4. mites

UBF   **50.** Tests commonly performed on CSF include

    1. total protein level determinations
    2. glucose level determinations
    3. chloride level determinations
    4. white blood cell counts

AP   **51.** Peristalsis is

1. the digestive system's method of absorption
2. a way to measure digestive capacity
3. part of the stomach
4. wavelike intestinal contractions that aid the movement of food

CPM   **52.** Strategic planning for a health care organization involves

1. daily operational planning
2. long-range planning
3. departmental budgeting
4. mission, goals, and objectives

CBC   **53.** Lipemic serum can be due to

1. ingestion of alcohol
2. bacterial contamination
3. excessive fasting
4. ingestion of fatty substances

AP   **54.** Laboratory testing of the muscular system includes which of the following analyses?

1. Clinical assays of kinase and lactate dehydrogenase
2. Microscopic examination
3. Analysis of autoimmune antibodies
4. Culturing of biopsy tissue

SDT   **55.** Specimens that require protection from light include those for

1. CBC, Diff, and platelet count
2. testing cold agglutinins and cryofibrinogen
3. glucose and cholesterol determinations
4. vitamin B_{12}, carotene, and folate determinations

HCS   **56.** In the clinical chemistry section, which of the following assays is (are) usually performed?

   1. Total proteins
   2. Triglycerides
   3. Cholesterol
   4. Cryofibrinogen

DIRECTIONS (Questions 57–69): Each of the questions or incomplete statements below is followed by suggested answers or completions. Select the **BEST** answer in each case.

VP   **57.** During a venipuncture procedure, a tourniquet should not be left on a patient more than

   A. 10 sec.
   B. 1 min.
   C. 3 min.
   D. 5 min.

BCE   **58.** The yellow-topped vacuum collection tube has which of the following additives?

   A. EDTA
   B. SST
   C. Trisodium citrate
   D. SPS

AE   **59.** Which of the following is the correct Spanish phrase for "How old are you?"

   A. Ya tomo el desayuno?
   B. Como se llama?
   C. Cuantos anos tiene usted?
   D. Entiende usted?

HCS   **60.** To become a medical technologist or clinical laboratory scientist requires which of the following educational degrees as a minimum?

      A. Associate's
      B. Bachelor's
      C. Master's
      D. Doctorate

ASC   **61.** *Postprandial* refers to

      A. 2-hr. fasting
      B. 12-hr. fasting
      C. after eating
      D. before eating

CBC   **62.** When hemoglobin is released and serum becomes tinged with pink or red, this condition is referred to as

      A. hemoconcentration
      B. hemophilia
      C. hemolysis
      D. lymphocytosis

BCE   **63.** Which of the following tests usually requires blood collected in a royal-blue-topped blood collection vacuum tube?

      A. Cortisol level
      B. CBC count
      C. Lactate dehydrogenase level
      D. Lead level

SPP   **64.** Which of the following should be used to decontaminate the site prior to skin puncture?

      A. Isopropanol
      B. Povidone-iodine
      C. Diluted chlorox
      D. Methanol

AP   **65.** What is the blood pH range in a normal human body?

      A. 0–7
      B. 6.5–10
      C. 7.35–7.45
      D. 7.55–8.45

HCS   **66.** The rapid plasma reagin (RPR) test is usually run in which of the following clinical laboratory sections?

      A. Clinical chemistry
      B. Clinical immunology
      C. Clinical microbiology
      D. Hematology

HCS   **67.** A primary consultant on drug therapy is

      A. an occupational therapist
      B. a physical therapist
      C. a pharmacist
      D. a laboratory supervisor

AE   **68.** A deciliter (dL) is equivalent to

      A. 1/2 liter
      B. 1/3 liter
      C. 1/10 liter
      D. 1/100 liter

LRI   **69.** Which of the following agencies maintains national surveillance of health care workers' accidental exposures?

    A. FDA
    B. JCAHO
    C. OSHA
    D. CDC

DIRECTIONS (Questions 70–100): For each of the following questions or incomplete statements, **ONE** or **MORE** of the numbered responses are correct. In each case, select

    A. if only 1, 2, and 3 are correct
    B. if only 1 and 3 are correct
    C. if only 2 and 4 are correct
    D. if only 4 is correct
    E. if all are correct

CPM   **70.** Imagine that a health care worker must collect a blood specimen from a hospitalized patient named Janie Doe. What is (are) the most appropriate way(s) to identify her?

    1. Ask: "Are you Ms. Janie Doe?"
    2. Ask: "What is your name?"
    3. Ask: "What is your identification number?"
    4. Check her hospital armband

TQM   **71.** Quality improvement efforts frequently involve monitoring

    1. the phlebotomist's technique
    2. the frequency of hematomas
    3. re-collection rates
    4. multiple sticks on the same patient

SDT   **72.** To chill a specimen as it is transported, the health care worker should use

    1. water
    2. refrigerated cooling elements
    3. small pieces or chips of ice
    4. frozen blocks of ice

SFA   **73.** Health care providers may encounter hazards from radiation exposure in the

    1. nuclear medicine department
    2. x-ray department
    3. radioimmunoassay section of the chemistry laboratory
    4. physical therapy department

IC   **74.** Which of the following make up the chain of infection that leads to nosocomial infections?

    1. Source
    2. Mode of transmission
    3. Susceptible host
    4. Susceptible vector

UBF   **75.** The O & P test is usually performed on

    1. urine
    2. whole blood
    3. seminal fluid
    4. feces

BCE   **76.** Which of the following is (are) assays used specifically to test thyroid function?

    1. TSH level
    2. T_4 level
    3. Thyroxine level
    4. Thrombin time

VP   **77.** If an inpatient does not have an identification bracelet, who should be asked to make the identification prior to a venipuncture?

1. A family member
2. The patient
3. The clerk who checked the patient in
4. The nurse in charge of the patient

AP   **78.** Homeostasis refers to

1. integumentary system
2. being chemically balanced
3. muscular system
4. steady state condition

LRI   **79.** NIDA defines

1. legal standards for venipuncture
2. educational standards
3. informed consent requirements for states
4. standards for collection and testing for substance abuse

CPM   **80.** Which of the following procedures require(s) exact timing for specimen collection?

1. Glucose tolerance tests
2. Therapeutic drug monitoring
3. 24-hr. urine samples
4. Bleeding-time tests

AP   **81.** *STDs* refer to

1. gonorrhea, genital herpes, syphilis
2. sexually transmitted diseases
3. human immunodeficiency virus (HIV)
4. hyperventilation episodes

CS   **82.** Which large artery or arteries carry blood to the body from the left side of the heart?

      1. Venae cavae
      2. Carotid
      3. Mesenteric
      4. Aortic

BCE   **83.** Which of the following would not typically be found on a microcollection tray?

      1. Disposable gloves
      2. Marking pens
      3. Lancets
      4. Needles for vacuum tubes and syringes

VP   **84.** The preferred position for a hospitalized patient during a venipuncture procedure is

      1. sitting
      2. reclining
      3. standing
      4. supine

ASC   **85.** Which of the following medications might interfere with the GTT?

      1. Clofibrate
      2. Corticosteroids
      3. Estrogens
      4. Diuretics

UBF   **86.** When the health care worker transports amniotic fluid to the laboratory, the specimen must be

1. protected from light
2. kept in a slurry of ice water
3. transported immediately
4. transported in a plastic vial

AP   **87.** DNA

1. is a double helix
2. is located in the nucleus
3. contains thousands of genes
4. is the same in all humans

BCE   **88.** Which of the following anticoagulant(s) is (are) used frequently for clinical cytogenetics blood studies?

1. Sodium citrate
2. Sodium oxalate
3. Ammonium oxalate
4. Sodium heparin

VP   **89.** The most common sites for venipuncture are the

1. median cubital vein
2. cephalic vein
3. basilic vein
4. femoral vein

CBC   **90.** Which of the following can affect laboratory tests on blood specimens?

1. Altitude
2. Temperature
3. Humidity
4. Geographic location

ASC **91.** Which of the following tests require(s) timed blood specimens?

    1. GTT
    2. Thyroxine
    3. Therapeutic drug monitoring
    4. Transferrin

AP **92.** The pharynx is best described by which of the following?

    1. Releases hormones for respiration
    2. Is a tubelike passageway
    3. Begins to absorb O_2 as it passes through to the lungs
    4. Allows for food and air to pass

BCE **93.** Which of the following laboratory procedures usually require(s) a blood smear?

    1. Blood cell count, differential
    2. Carcinoembryonic antigen (CEA)
    3. Heinz bodies special stain
    4. Chloramphenicol

BCE **94.** The term A/G ratio refers to which of the following proteins?

    1. Alpha-fibrinogen
    2. Albumin
    3. Gamma-transpeptidase
    4. Globulin

LRI **95.** The ideal risk management model deals with

    1. education of employees, patients, and visitors
    2. risk identification and analysis
    3. risk treatment to prevent harm
    4. risk transfer and risk evaluation

AP   **96.** Disorders of the respiratory system include which of the following?

    1. Tuberculosis, laryngitis, bronchitis, whooping cough
    2. Pneumonia, influenza, asthma, emphysema, cystic fibrosis
    3. Tumors
    4. Ulcers

BCE   **97.** Criterion (criteria) used to describe vacuum collection tube size is (are)

    1. external tube diameter
    2. external tube length
    3. maximum amount of specimen to be drawn
    4. internal tube diameter

CBC   **98.** The word *nonfasting* should be indicated on the specimen or requisition form if the patient

    1. did not have breakfast
    2. ate breakfast
    3. needs a blood glucose level determination
    4. ate a small snack

PP   **99.** Complications resulting from multiple deep skin punctures on an infant's heel include

    1. hepatitis
    2. AIDS
    3. pneumonia
    4. osteomyelitis

HHB   **100.** Which of the following blood assays can assist in the diagnosis and evaluation of anemia?

    1. Hemoglobin
    2. Na$^+$
    3. Hematocrit
    4. Methemalbumin

Practice Test Questions 3

Answers and Discussion

Page numbers refer to Garza D, Becan-McBride K: *Phlebotomy Handbook, 4th ed.* Stamford, CT, Appleton & Lange, 1996.

1. **(D)** *(p. 527)*

2. **(E)** Confidential patient information and materials include the patient's verbal statements, laboratory test results, conversations between the physician and the patient, and employee drug testing reports. *(p. 496)*

3. **(C)** For a 24-hr. urine collection, the patient should be advised to void at 7:00 AM and discard the urine, then collect all urine for the next 24 hr. in the special container provided. The patient should be cautioned that to have good results, *all* the urine must be saved or the procedure will have to be repeated. *(p. 468)*

4. **(B)** A tachometer indicates speed in revolutions per minute (RPM). *(p. 461)*

5. **(E)** PROs use documentation in the medical records to evaluate the quality of care, medical stability of patients, necessity of tests and procedures, adequacy of discharge planning, and occurrence of avoidable discomfort or death. PROs can impose fines, impose sanctions, or deny reimbursement for care if patient care is inappropriate. *(p. 404)*

6. **(E)** The integumentary system consists of skin, hair, sweat and oil glands, teeth, and fingernails. *(p. 45)*

7. **(A)** Skin prevents water loss and allows for perspiration as needed by the body during exercise, fever, or weather conditions. Sebaceous glands in the skin produce oils for skin and hair protection. *(p. 45)*

8. **(B)** Key points in all negligence cases include duty and breach of duty and proximate causation and damages. *(p. 496)*

9. **(E)** The Isostat system is a special blood culture tube system that has (1) lysing and anticoagulating agents, (2) reagents in the tube that inactivate HIV, and (3) containment adapters that help protect phlebotomists and laboratorians against infection due to aerosol spray or breakage during centrifugation. *(pp. 275–276)*

10. **(E)** Requisitions should contain the following information: patient's full name, patient's identification number, patient's date of birth, types of tests to be performed, dates of tests, patient's room number and bed assignment, physician's name and code, test status (time, stat, fasting), billing information (optional), and special precautions. *(p. 160)*

11. **(B)** Blood tests to detect syphilis are the RPR test and the VDRL test. *(pp. 120–121)*

12. **(B)** The two upper chambers of the heart are the right and left atria. The singular spelling is *atrium*. *(p. 79)*

13 **(B)** Melanin provides skin color and protects underlying tissues from absorbing ultraviolet rays from the sun. *(p. 45)*

14. **(A)** Blood collected for an electrolyte panel is usually tested for sodium, potassium, bicarbonate, and chloride. *(p. 22)*

15. **(D)** *(p. 528)*

16. **(B)** Disclosure of confidential information can result in a breach of the patient's rights and an invasion of the patient's privacy. *(p. 416)*

17. **(E)** Multipurpose (ABC) fire extinguishers can be used for all the listed types of fires. *(p. 385)*

18. **(A)** Good technique in hand washing for the prevention of disease transmission in hospitals involves warm running water, soap, and friction. *(p. 366)*

19. **(A)** Protein, bilirubin, and hemoglobin analysis are part of the chemical anlysis in a routine urinalysis. *(p. 322)*

20. **(E)** *On-site testing, alternate-site testing, near-patient testing,* and *patient-focused testing* are terms synonymous with *point-of-care testing. (p. 306)*

21. **(A)** Blood glucose levels are determined for patients having any of the following tests performed: (1) glucagon tolerance test, (2) epinephrine tolerance test, and (3) lactose tolerance test. *(pp. 282–283)*

22. **(B)** Both the endocrine system and the nervous system function for communication, control, and integration of bodily functions. *(pp. 51, 62)*

23. **(B)** A C&S test is a culture and sensitivity test performed in clinical microbiology. This test involves culturing and identifying bacterial pathogens and testing for inhibition of bacterial growth by an antibiotic. *(pp. 26–27)*

24. **(A)** The four chambers of the heart are the right and left atria and the right and left ventricles. They perform the pumping action of the heart to push blood throughout the body. *(p. 79)*

25. **(A)** Equipment required for the scalp vein venipuncture includes a 23- or 25-gauge winged infusion set; a large, flat rubber band; and a disposable razor. *(p. 249)*

26. **(D)** The evacuated tube method for venipuncture requires a double-pointed multiple-sample needle. *(pp. 127, 174)*

27. **(B)** No anticoagulant is found in the royal-blue-topped blood collection vacuum tube. *(p. 122)*

28. (A) *(p. 526)*

29. (A) The FDA evaluates the safety, clinical efficacy, and medical efficacy of the equipment and supplies used in blood collection. *(p. 510)*

30. (B) Continuous quality improvement (CQI) refers to the improvement of health care structures, processes, and outcomes, and client satisfaction. Quality control (QC) procedures refer to monitoring only processes. *(pp. 450, 452)*

31. (D) The average person inhales and exhales about 15 times per minute, or about 20,000 times per day. During the normal process of respiration, the exchange of carbon dioxide and oxygen takes place. *(pp. 52–53)*

32. (A) Systole is the contraction phase of the heart rhythm; diastole is the relaxation phase of the heart rhythm. *(p. 80)*

33. (C) Falsely decreased values of a blood analyte can be mistakenly interpreted as normal or subnormal if the blood analyte is truly in an elevated range or a normal range, respectively. *(p. 214)*

34. (B) Warming the site prior to skin puncture will increase blood flow to the site. *(p. 195)*

35. (B) The most efficient and accurate specimen labels are those that are generated by a hospital (or laboratory) computer system. Computers can generate enough labels containing all the appropriate patient identification criteria for each tube required to be collected. The labels also indicate the specific tests requested, the color of tube required, and unique accession numbers or sample numbers to be used for that particular collection time. Bar codes can also be used on the specimen labels, which are then automatically read by laboratory instruments. Computerization of the collection process can significantly decrease errors. *(pp. 425–426)*

36. (C) The butterfly needle is the most commonly used intravenous device that is sometimes used in the collection of blood from patients who are difficult to stick by conventional methods. *(pp. 127, 169)*

37. (A) The largest group of nongovernmental hospitals is referred to as community hospitals. *(p. 9)*

38. (B) The department of electrocardiography is used as a diagnostic service to record the electric current produced by the contractions of the heart muscle. *(p. 15)*

39. (B) Sensory neurons (nerve cells) transmit impulses from muscle tissues to the brain or spinal cord. Motor neurons transmit impulses to muscles from the spinal cord or brain. *(p. 51)*

40. (E) Specimens that may require chilling include those for gastrin, ammonia, lactic acid, renin, catecholamines, parathyroid hormone, PT, PTT, glucagon, and blood gas analysis. *(p. 427)*

41. (D) Sodium citrate is used frequently in coagulation blood studies. *(p. 122)*

42. (C) Plasma is the fluid portion of the blood and is obtained by mixing the blood with an anticoagulant that prevents it from clotting. *(p. 78)*

43. (A) The kidney's main function is to regulate the amount of water, electrolytes (sodium, potassium, chloride), and nitrogenous wastes in the body. *(p. 58)*

44. (C) The clinical laboratory department is composed of two major areas: clinical pathology and anatomic pathology. *(p. 16)*

45. (B) *(p. 527)*

46. (E) Outcome assessments for quality improvement may involve evaluating recovery rates, cure rates, nosocomial infection rates, and return-to-normal-function rates. *(p. 452)*

47. (A) Positive body language can include the following: maintaining erect posture; smiling; making eye contact; having relaxed hands, arms, and shoulders; communicating face to face; communicating at eye level; displaying good grooming habits; and maintaining an appropriate zone of comfort. *(p. 472)*

48. (B) EPA and OSHA regulations, as well as state and local laws, regulate the disposal of wastes. *(p. 381)*

49. (C) Mosquitoes and mites act as vectors in transmitting infectious diseases. *(p. 350)*

50. (E) Total protein, glucose, chloride, and white blood cell count analyses are commonly performed on CSF. *(p. 328)*

51. (D) Peristalsis consists of wavelike intestinal contractions that aid the movement of food through the intestinal tract. *(p. 56)*

52. (C) Strategic planning for a health care organization involves long-range planning in accordance with the organization's mission, goals, and objectives. *(p. 485)*

53. (D) Lipemic serum can be due to ingestion of fatty substances. *(p. 211)*

54. (E) Laboratory testing of the muscular system could include assays of specific muscle enzymes such as creatine phosphokinase and lactate dehydrogenase, analysis of autoimmune antibodies, microscopic examination, or culturing of muscle biopsy tissue. *(p. 51)*

55. (D) Specimens that require protection from light include those for vitamin B_{12}, carotene, and folate determinations. *(p. 427)*

56. (A) In the clinical chemistry section, total protein, triglycerides, and cholesterol assays are usually run. *(p. 22)*

57. (B) A tourniquet should not be left on the patient's arm for more than 1 min. *(p. 170)*

58. (D) Sodium polyanetholesulfonate (SPS) is the additive in the vacuum tube with the yellow top. *(p. 103)*

59. (C) *(p. 526)*

60. (B) The medical technologist (MT) has a minimum of a bachelor's degree in a biological science. *(p. 20)*

61. (C) *Postprandial* means after eating. *(pp. 281–282)*

62. (C) Hemolysis is when the RBCs are lysed and release hemoglobin. *(pp. 208–209)*

63. (D) The lead assay requires blood collected in a royal-blue-topped blood collection vacuum tube. *(pp. 116, 122)*

64. (A) Isopropanol should be used to decontaminate the skin puncture site. Povidone-iodine is not recommended for the skin puncture site because it can falsely elevate potassium, phosphorus, and uric acid determinations. *(p. 197)*

65. (C) The blood pH of a normal human body has a narrow range of between 7.35 and 7.45. Deviations from the normal, or reference, range can be dangerous and deadly. *(p. 55)*

66. (B) Personnel in the clinical immunology section run procedures to determine antigen-antibody reactions. The RPR assay is run to test for syphilis. *(p. 27)*

67. (C) The pharmacist is involved with members of the health care team as a primary consultant on drug therapy. *(p. 15)*

68. (C) *(p. 527)*

69. (D) The CDC maintains national surveillance of health care workers' accidental exposure. *(p. 498)*

70. (C) The most appropriate way to identify Ms. Doe is to ask, "What is your name?" and to check her hospital armband. *(p. 467)*

71. (E) Quality improvement efforts frequently involve monitoring the following: the phlebotomist's technique, the frequency of hematomas, re-collection rates, and multiple sticks on the same patient. All of these issues can potentially result in a negative outcome for the patient. *(p. 453)*

72. (B) It is best to use ice water to chill a specimen during transport to the testing laboratory. Solid chunks of ice should not be used because the specimen may freeze. Freezing cells causes hemolysis. *(p. 427)*

73. (A) Health care providers may encounter hazards from radiation exposure in the nuclear medicine and x-ray departments and in the radioimmunoassay section of the chemistry laboratory. *(pp. 387–388)*

74. (A) The three components that make up the chain of infection that leads to nosocomial infections are (1) source, (2) mode of transmission, and (3) susceptible host. *(p. 347)*

75. (D) The O & P test is usually performed on feces. *(p. 328)*

76. (A) Thyroid-stimulating hormone (TSH) and thyroxine (T_4) level determinations are procedures specifically for testing thyroid function. *(p. 120)*

77. (D) The nurse in charge of the patient should be asked to make the identification if the patient does not have a hospital armband or bracelet. *(p. 159)*

78. (C) *Homeostasis* refers to a steady-state, or chemically balanced, condition in the body. *(p. 43)*

79. (D) NIDA defines requirements for specimen collection, processing, analysis, and reporting of results for substance abuse testing. *(pp. 500–501)*

80. (E) The following procedures require exact timing for specimen collection: glucose tolerance tests, therapeutic drug monitoring, 24-hr. urine samples, and bleeding-time tests. *(p. 468)*

81. (A) Sexually transmitted diseases (STDs) include gonorrhea, genital herpes, syphilis, and human immunodeficiency virus (HIV). *(p. 60)*

82. (D) The aorta is the largest artery and carries blood to the entire body. *(p. 82)*

83. (D) Needles for vacuum tubes and syringes are not needed on a microcollection tray. *(p. 145)*

84. (C) A reclining, or supine, position is the *preferred* position for a patient during venipuncture. However, sitting in a sturdy chair with arm supports is also acceptable. *(pp. 165, 167)*

85. **(E)**   Clofibrate, cortocosteroids, diuretics, and estrogens all can interfere with GTT results. *(pp. 277–278)*

86. **(B)**   Amniotic fluid should be transported to the laboratory immediately after collection and should be protected from light during transportation. *(p. 330)*

87. **(A)**   DNA is described as a *double helix* or *twisted ladder.* It is located in the nucleus and contains thousands of genes. It is not the same in all individuals since it contains codes for the individual's genetic makeup. *(p. 43)*

88. **(D)**   Sodium heparin is used for clinical cytogenetics studies. *(p. 122)*

89. **(A)**   The most common sites for venipuncture are the median cubital, cephalic, and basilic veins because they lie close to the surface of the skin and are most prominent. *(p. 167)*

90. **(E)**   Altitude, temperature, humidity, and geographic location can all affect laboratory tests on blood specimens. *(p. 213)*

91. **(B)**   The glucose tolerance test (GTT) and therapeutic drug monitoring require timed blood specimens. *(pp. 281, 284)*

92. **(C)**   The pharnyx is a tubelike passageway for food and air. Along with the larynx (voice box), it determines the quality of voice. *(pp. 53–54)*

93. **(B)**   The blood cell count including the differential and the Heinz bodies special stain usually require a blood smear. *(pp. 111, 121)*

94. **(C)**   The term *A/G ratio* refers to the albumin/globulin ratio. *(pp. 118, 121)*

95. *(E)*   The components of an ideal risk management model include education of employees, patients, and visitors; risk identification and analysis; risk treatment to prevent harm; and risk transfer and risk evaluation. *(p. 512)*

96. *(A)* Disorders of the respiratory system include tuberculosis, laryngitis, bronchitis, whooping cough, pneumonia, influenza, asthma, emphysema, cystic fibrosis, and tumors. *(p. 56)*

97. **(A)** The external tube diameter and length plus the maximum amount of specimen to be collected into the vacuum tube are the criteria used to describe vacuum collection tube size. *(p. 101)*

98. **(C)** The word *nonfasting* should be indicated on the specimen or requisition form if the patient ate breakfast or even a small snack. *(p. 210)*

99. **(D)** Osteomyelitis can result from multiple deep skin punctures on an infant's heel. *(p. 241)*

100. **(B)** Hemoglobin and hematocrit determinations are two blood assays that can assist in the diagnosis and evaluation of anemia. *(p. 315)*

Practice Test Questions 4

DIRECTIONS (Questions 1–20): For each of the following questions or incomplete statements, **ONE** or **MORE** of the numbered responses are correct. In each case, select

    A. if only 1, 2, and 3 are correct
    B. if only 1 and 3 are correct
    C. if only 2 and 4 are correct
    D. if only 4 is correct
    E. if all are correct

SPP   **1.** Preferred skin puncture sites are the

    1. second and fourth fingers
    2. thumb
    3. middle, or third, finger
    4. fifth, or pinky, finger

PP   **2.** Equipment for skin puncture on children and infants includes

    1. sterile automatic pediatric lancet device, disposable
    2. 70% isopropyl alcohol swab in a sterile package
    3. Microtainer (Becton Dickinson VACUTAINER Systems, Franklin Lakes, NJ)
    4. 23- or 25-gauge winged infusion set

ASC   **3.** A false-negative blood culture is more likely to occur if

  1. iodine is not wiped from the tops of the blood culture tubes
  2. the indwelling catheter is used to obtain the culture specimen
  3. too little blood is used for the culture
  4. the health care worker palpates the venipuncture site after the site has been prepared without first cleaning the gloved finger

HHB   **4.** Which of the following problems should be avoided in POC glucose testing?

  1. Specimen is collected at wrong time
  2. Reagents are outdated
  3. Wrong volume of specimen is collected
  4. Calibrators are not properly used

IC   **5.** Which of the following commonly identified pathogenic microorganisms cause(s) nosocomial infections of the ear?

  1. *Pseudomonas aeruginosa*
  2. *Streptococcus pneumoniae*
  3. Gram-negative bacilli
  4. *Moraxella lacunata*

AE   **6.** The abbreviation QNS refers to

  1. quality not satisfactory
  2. quantitatively not sound
  3. quantity normally superior
  4. quantity not sufficient

ASC   **7.** Which of the following is (are) used for bleeding-time tests?

     1. Isostat system
     2. Surgicutt
     3. Thrombin time
     4. Simplate R

LRI   **8.** The relationship between a physician and a patient is a contractual one in the legal sense. What are the basic elements of this type of contract?

     1. The physician offers to provide a service to the patient
     2. The patient uses the service for disease treatment
     3. The patient accepts and pays for the treatment
     4. The patient signs a contract

IC   **9.** The actual occurrence of an infection from a biohazardous specimen depends on the

     1. virulence of a host
     2. virulence of the infecting agent
     3. susceptibility of the infecting agent
     4. host's susceptibility

AP   **10.** The anterior, or ventral, surface of the body is separated into which of the following body cavities?

     1. Thoracic
     2. Abdominal
     3. Pelvic
     4. Cranial

BCE   **11.** Which of the following statements apply to the B-D Unopette?

     1. It has a plastic reservoir containing a premeasured volume of reagent for diluting
     2. It has a reusable, self-filling diluting pipette
     3. It consists of a straight, thin-walled, uniform-bore, glass capillary tube fitted into a plastic holder
     4. It is a blade-retraction mechanism

AP   **12.** Germ cells are defined as

     1. sperm
     2. neurons
     3. ova
     4. hair follicles

SPP   **13.** Prior to a skin puncture procedure, the phlebotomist should

     1. prepare him- or herself emotionally
     2. prepare all supplies and equipment needed
     3. put on clean gloves
     4. talk to the patient's physician

HHB   **14.** Which of the following instruments can run glucose tests on arterial, capillary, or venous whole blood samples?

     1. I-STAT
     2. AccuMeter
     3. Nova Biomedical Stat Profile Analyzer (Nova Biomedical, Waltham, MA)
     4. HemoCue β-Glucose Analyzer (HemoCue, Inc., Mission Viejo, CA)

IC   **15.** Which of the following diseases usually require(s) strict, or complete, isolation?

1. Anthrax
2. *Vibrio* infection
3. Rabies
4. *Salmonella* infection

TQM   **16.** Health care workers who perform phlebotomy procedures are often asked to maintain the quality control and preventive maintenance records on which of the following types of equipment?

1. Thermometers
2. Sphygmomanometers
3. Centrifuges
4. Blood pressure cuff

CPM   **17.** A health care worker's first steps after entering a patient's hospital room to perform a venipuncture should include which of the following?

1. Introduce him- or herself
2. Identify him- or herself as a part of the hospital or laboratory staff
3. Provide information as to the purpose of the visit
4. Indicate to the patient that the venipuncture will not hurt

LRI   **18.** A medical expert witness

1. witnessed the event or occurrence in question
2. must testify about professional standards of care
3. must support the physicians in court
4. must be knowledgeable about medical practice patterns

SDT   **19.** Specimens that require warming to body temperature are those for

     1. CBC, Diff, and platelet count
     2. vitamin B_{12}, carotene, and folate determinations
     3. glucose and cholesterol determinations
     4. testing cold agglutinins and cryofibrinogen

SFA   **20.** Radiation exposure can be minimized by

     1. staying as far away from the radiation as possible
     2. using lead shielding
     3. limiting the time of exposure
     4. avoiding the sight of the emitting radiation source

DIRECTIONS (Questions 21–61): Each of the questions or incomplete statements below is followed by suggested answers or completions. Select the **BEST** answer in each case.

ASC   **21.** For the Surgicutt bleeding-time test, the blood pressure cuff must be inflated on the patient's upper arm to

     A. 20 mm Hg
     B. 30 mm Hg
     C. 40 mm Hg
     D. 60 mm Hg

PP   **22.** Which of the following venous areas is most accessible and chosen for venipuncture for most toddlers and children?

     A. Dorsal hand
     B. Femoral
     C. Antecubital fossa
     D. Anterior wrist

CBC   **23.** Which of the following blood analytes is affected by diurnal rhythm?

       A. Cortisol
       B. BUN
       C. Creatinine
       D. CK

BCE   **24.** A blood cell count requires whole blood collected in a

       A. green-topped tube
       B. purple-topped tube
       C. gray-topped tube
       D. light-blue-topped tube

CS   **25.** Serum is blood

       A. that is highly oxygenated
       B. containing anticoagulants
       C. without anticoagulants
       D. rich in carbon monoxide

HCS   **26.** What is the principal task of the clinical chemistry section?

       A. Providing blood products to patients
       B. Providing a detailed study of individual chromosomes
       C. Culturing and identifying bacterial pathogens
       D. Running toxicology and hormone assays

VP   **27.** When the evacuated tube method is used for venipuncture, which is the correct order of collection for the following tubes: blood culture tubes, coagulation tube, and hematology tube? The tubes with the

      A. light-blue top, lavender top, yellow blood culture tubes
      B. lavender top, light-blue top, yellow blood culture tubes
      C. yellow blood culture tubes, blue top, lavender top
      D. light-blue top, yellow blood culture tubes, lavender top

SPP   **28.** *Osteomyelitis* is

      A. infection of the blood
      B. infection of the spinal fluid
      C. inflammation and infection of the bone
      D. inflammation of the finger

PP   **29.** After a dorsal hand vein blood collection, pressure should be applied over the venipuncture site with a dry gauze sponge for

      A. 20–30 sec.
      B. 30–60 sec.
      C. 1/2–1½ min.
      D. 2–3 min.

SDT   **30.** Serum should be transported to the laboratory for testing and separated from blood cells within which of the following time periods to prevent erroneous test results?

      A. 5 hr.
      B. 4 hr.
      C. 2 hr.
      D. 5 min.

CPM **31.** "Nothing by mouth" means that

    A. intravenous fluids are being administered
    B. the patient has been fasting
    C. the patient's temperature should not be taken by mouth
    D. the patient cannot chew solid foods

AE **32.** How is the phrase "Do you understand?" expressed in Spanish?

    A. Como se llama?
    B. Entiende usted?
    C. Su domicilio?
    D. Quien es su doctor?

BCE **33.** *Sedimentation rate* is abbreviated

    A. PNH
    B. ESR
    C. BUN
    D. AST

CS **34.** Blood that is returning to the right side of the heart from the body is transported by which of the following veins?

    A. Coronary vein
    B. Portal vein
    C. Inferior vena cava
    D. Aorta

AP **35.** An XX pair of chromosomes means that the fetus will be

    A. a baby boy
    B. a baby girl
    C. a brown-haired child
    D. a blue-eyed baby

HCS 36. Which of the following laboratory sections usually has a toxicology area?

A. Clinical microbiology
B. Cytogenetics
C. Clinical serology
D. Clinical chemistry

BCE 37. Which of the following is frequently used in the micro-collection of electrolytes and general chemistry blood specimens?

A. B-D Unopette
B. Monoject Corvac tube
C. Heparinized Natelson tube
D. B-D Microtainer

AE 38. For hematology calculations, the MCV is equivalent to

A. hematocrit × 100
B. hemoglobin × 10
C. MCH expressed in picograms
D. hematocrit × 10/RBC count in millions

TQM 39. Cause-and-effect diagrams are used in quality improvement methodologies and are designed to assist with

A. making bar charts that show the frequency of problems
B. identifying interactions between people, methods, equipment, supplies, and/or reagents
C. stimulating creative ideas
D. breaking out components into a flowchart

SFA   **40.** If a health care provider is in an area of the health care facility where a fire starts, she/he should first

    A. attempt to extinguish the fire, using the proper extinguisher
    B. pull the lever in the fire alarm box
    C. close all the doors and windows before leaving the area
    D. block the entrances so that others will not enter the fire area

UBF   **41.** The first analyte that can be detected in urine or serum produced in pregnancy is

    A. PRL
    B. HCG
    C. ACTH
    D. TSH

HCS   **42.** Which of the following best describes a responsibility of technical supervisors of clinical laboratory sections?

    A. Performs various chemical, microscopic, microbiological, or immunologic tests pertaining to patient care and diagnosis
    B. Prepares specimens for reference laboratories
    C. Prepares daily work schedules to provide adequate coverage and effective use of personnel
    D. Collects adequate and correct blood specimens by venipuncture or microcollection from adults, children, and infants

AP   **43.** Cell metabolism involves energy production by which of the following processes?

    A. DNA transfer
    B. Perspiration
    C. Breaking down chemical substances
    D. Hemolysis

CS   **44.** A *differential count* refers to

        A. blood pressure
        B. contraction of the heart
        C. enumeration of specific types of WBCs
        D. a heart murmur

CS   **45.** The hepatic artery delivers blood to the

        A. liver
        B. heart
        C. legs and lower trunk
        D. arms

AE   **46.** Which of the following is the correct phrase in Spanish for "Have you been here before?"

        A. Entiende usted?
        B. Su domicilio?
        C. Quien es su doctor?
        D. Ha estado usted aqui antes?

IC   **47.** Disinfectants are

        A. chemicals used to inhibit the growth and development of microorganisms but do not necessarily kill them
        B. used frequently on skin
        C. chemicals used to remove or kill pathogenic microorganisms
        D. quaternary ammonium compounds

UBF   **48.** Pericardial fluid is collected from the

        A. abdomen
        B. sac around the heart
        C. joints
        D. sac around the lungs

BCE   **49.** A prefilled device used as a collection and dilution unit is the

    A. B-D Unopette
    B. Monoject Corvac tube
    C. heparinized Natelson tube
    D. AVL microtainer

CS   **50.** Universal donors are individuals with blood type

    A. A
    B. B
    C. AB
    D. O

AP   **51.** How many lungs do normal humans have?

    A. 2
    B. 3
    C. 4
    D. 5

BCE   **52.** The Autolet II Clinisafe (Ulster Scientific, Inc., New Paltz, NY) is a

    A. safety device for collecting arterial blood gas specimens
    B. safety device for collecting specimens by venipuncture
    C. safe method to dispose of sharps
    D. spring-activated puncture device for collecting capillary blood

HCS   **53.** Which of the following assays is performed in the immunohematology sections?

        A. Chromosomal analysis
        B. Proteus OX agglutinins
        C. Direct Coombs' test
        D. Ketones

CBC   **54.** Which of the following blood analyte levels increases with age?

        A. Estrogen
        B. Cholesterol
        C. Growth hormone
        D. Glucose

BCE   **55.** Figure 4-1 shows

        A. Samplette capillary blood collectors
        B. B-D Unopettes
        C. B-D Microtainer
        D. Monoject Corvac tubes

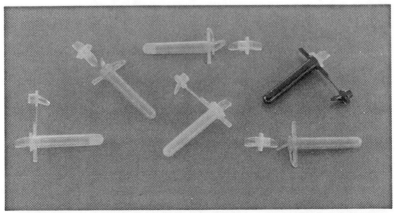

Figure 4-1 *(Courtesy of Sherwood Davis & Geck, St. Louis, MO.)*

ASC   **56.** To obtain the blood trough level for a medication, the patient's blood should be collected

    A. immediately after administration of the medication
    B. immediately prior to administration of the medication
    C. 2 hr. prior to administration of the medication
    D. 2 hr. after administration of the medication

UBF   **57.** For the urinary pregnancy test, the preferred urine specimen is a

    A. 2-hr. urine collection
    B. 24-hr. urine sample
    C. random urine sample
    D. clean-catch midstream sample

HHB   **58.** Tolerance limits for a quality control chart are determined from data obtained for how many days?

    A. 10
    B. 20
    C. 30
    D. 35

CBC   **59.** Falsely increased laboratory results for a blood analyte can be

    A. caused by a medication competing with the blood analyte for a chromogenic reagent, thus falsely decreasing the resultant color of the reaction
    B. mistakenly interpreted as elevated or normal if the blood analyte is truly in a normal range or a decreased range, respectively
    C. mistakenly interpreted as normal or subnormal if the blood analyte is truly in an elevated range or a normal range, respectively
    D. both a and c

BCE **60.** The containers shown in Figure 4-2 were manufactured to be used for

    A. evacuated blood collection tubes
    B. tourniquets
    C. needles
    D. Monoject Corvac tubes

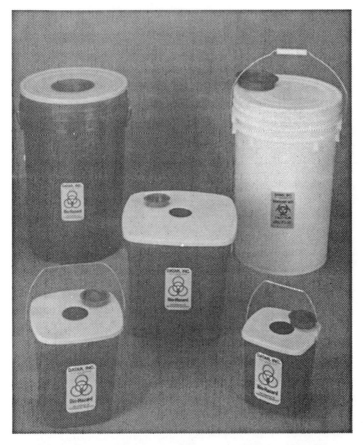

Figure 4-2 *(Courtesy of Datar, Inc., Long Lake, MN.)*

BCE   **61.** The health care worker should not use gloves with talc powder when collecting blood because the tubes of blood may become contaminated with this powder and result in falsely

    A. decreased iron values
    B. elevated TIBC values
    C. elevated copper values
    D. elevated calcium values

DIRECTIONS (Questions 62–91): For each of the following questions or incomplete statements, **ONE** or **MORE** of the numbered responses are correct. In each case, select

    A. if only 1, 2, and 3 are correct
    B. if only 1 and 3 are correct
    C. if only 2 and 4 are correct
    D. if only 4 is correct
    E. if all are correct

CPM   **62.** With therapeutic drug monitoring, the physician must have information that might include

    1. the time and date of collection
    2. whether the blood was collected before or after drug administration
    3. the length of infusion time
    4. the patient's fasting status

LRI   **63.** The basic purpose(s) of the medical record is (are) to

    1. allow for continuity of the patient's care plan
    2. document the patient's illness and treatment
    3. document communication between the physician and other members of the health care team
    4. provide a legal document for patients, the hospital, and employees

SPP **64.** Labeled skin puncture specimens should include the

  1. patient's name and identification number
  2. time of collection
  3. phlebotomist's initials
  4. date of collection

VP **65.** Reasons for not using arm veins for venipuncture include which of the following?

  1. The patient has IV lines in both arms
  2. The patient is burned
  3. The patient has casts on both arms
  4. The patient has edematous arms

BCE **66.** For which of the following assays should serum be obtained in a speckled-topped collection tube?

  1. Transaminase level
  2. Testosterone level
  3. Rubella determination
  4. Zinc level

CS **67.** Tests for blood types and cross-match testing for donor blood are done in which of the following areas of the laboratory?

  1. Hematology
  2. Immunohematology
  3. Clinical chemistry
  4. Blood bank

AP   **68.** The digestive system functions to

1. break down food chemically and physically into nutrients
2. secrete hormones for regulatory functions
3. eliminate the waste products of digestion
4. transport O_2 and CO_2

CBC   **69.** Which of the following can affect laboratory test results by leading to falsely elevated or decreased results?

1. Sneezing
2. Violent crying
3. Smiling
4. Medications

ASC   **70.** Which of the following condition(s) should the patient report to his/her physician before the GTT, since the condition(s) may affect the results of the GTT?

1. Hyperthyroidism
2. Pregnancy
3. Adrenal insufficiency
4. Acute pancreatitis

CPM   **71.** Basic responsibilities of health care managers or supervisors include

1. evaluating technical performance
2. measuring turnaround times
3. monitoring the budget and expenses
4. scheduling work hours

LRI   **72.** Malpractice cases typically have which of the following characteristics?

      1. The plaintiff believes that the health care provider did something wrong
      2. The plaintiff was injured
      3. The health care provider failed to use professional standards of care
      4. Damage was physical, mental, or financial

AP   **73.** Characteristics of the normal human body include which of the following?

      1. A backbone
      2. Bisymmetry
      3. Cavities for organs
      4. 11 organ systems

BCE   **74.** Gray-topped blood collection tubes can be ordered containing

      1. heparin
      2. potassium oxalate
      3. sodium citrate and thymol
      4. potassium oxalate and sodium fluoride

AP   **75.** The sagittal plane of the body

      1. runs lengthwise from front to back
      2. runs crosswise
      3. divides the body into right and left halves
      4. divides the body into upper and lower sections

BCE   **76.** For which of the following assays must blood be collected in a green-topped blood collection tube?

     1. Ammonia level
     2. Chromosomal analysis
     3. Cryofibrinogen level
     4. LE cell test

VP   **77.** If arm veins cannot be used for venipuncture, the preferred alternative veins lie in the

     1. ankles
     2. anterior surface of the wrist
     3. feet
     4. posterior surface of the wrist

SPP   **78.** Which of the following conditions has (have) an adverse effect on the quality of a finger stick?

     1. Swollen fingers
     2. Excessive milking of the finger
     3. Using the first drop of blood
     4. The presence of a wedding ring

CBC   **79.** During the blood collection process, which of the following actions can cause hemolysis?

     1. Slowly inverting the specimen tube by mixing
     2. Forcing blood into an evacuated collection tube from a syringe
     3. Using a butterfly needle for a venipuncture
     4. Vigorously shaking the specimen tube

ASC   **80.** Figure 4-3 shows swabbing of the arm in concentric circles in preparation of collecting blood for

     1. therapeutic drug monitoring
     2. blood cultures
     3. the lactose tolerance test
     4. blood donation

AP   **81.** Components of the respiratory system include the

     1. nose
     2. trachea
     3. lungs
     4. humerus

BCE   **82.** Which of the following is (are) true concerning the volume of plasma or serum that can generally be collected from a patient?

     1. 100–150 μL of plasma or serum can usually be collected from a premature infant
     2. 200–300 μL of plasma or serum can usually be collected from a full-term newborn
     3. Volumes larger than 300 μL of plasma or serum can usually be collected from an adult
     4. Only 300 μL of plasma or serum can usually be collected from a child

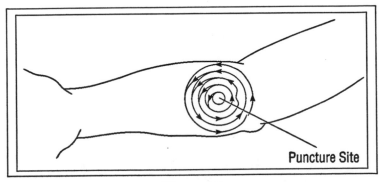

Figure 4-3

VP   **83.** Which of the following must be included on the label of the blood specimen or body fluid specimen?

    1. Patient's name
    2. Patient's identification number (if hospital patient)
    3. Time at which specimen was collected
    4. Attending physician's name

SPP   **84.** Which of the following sites is (are) **NOT** suitable for skin puncture?

    1. Finger
    2. Ankle and wrist
    3. Heel
    4. Toe

CBC   **85.** Which of the following circumstances usually result(s) in failure to collect blood during venipuncture?

    1. Needle is inserted through the vein
    2. Vacuum in the specimen is lost
    3. Veins are sclerosed
    4. Tourniquet is too tight

ASC   **86.** The use of gel serum separator tubes leads to falsely low blood levels for which of the following drugs?

    1. Lidocaine
    2. Phenytoin
    3. Pentobarbital
    4. Nicotine

LRI   **87.** Which of the following may be considered part of "discovery" in a blood collection lawsuit?

       1. Infection control logs and reports
       2. JCAHO standards
       3. Laboratory policies and procedures
       4. Board certification

CPM   **88.** Staffing for phlebotomy services involves

       1. recruitment, selection, placement, training
       2. keeping an inventory of supplies
       3. scheduling, compensation, evaluation
       4. clerical charting function

TQM   **89.** Westgard and his colleagues suggest a "5 Q" framework for clinical laboratories that focuses on

       1. quality planning and quality laboratory practices
       2. quality control of processes and quality assessment
       3. quality improvement
       4. quality expansion

SDT   **90.** Laboratory reports may be released to appropriate personnel by means of

       1. verbal reports
       2. computerized reports
       3. facsimile reports
       4. the patient

IC   **91.** Which of the following can lead to a laboratory-acquired infection?

       1. Drinking a soda in the specimen collection area
       2. Popping the cap off a vacuum blood collection tube
       3. Sustaining scratches from needles
       4. Rubbing the eyes in the specimen collection area

DIRECTIONS (Questions 92–100): Each of the questions or incomplete statements below is followed by suggested answers or completions. Select the **BEST** answer in each case.

ASC   **92.** Which of the following tests requires numerous blood collections?

       A. Arterial blood gas analysis
       B. GTT
       C. Aldosterone
       D. Drug screening

CS   **93.** Which arteries feed the head and neck regions?

       A. Hepatic
       B. Subclavian
       C. Brachial
       D. Carotid

AP   **94.** Glycogen is best defined as

       A. a substance for aiding digestion
       B. a hormone produced in the adrenals
       C. a hormone used for cell division
       D. stored glucose in muscles

HSC   **95.** The health care that is given to maintain and monitor normal health and to prevent diseases through immunizations is referred to as

       A. primary care
       B. secondary care
       C. tertiary care
       D. quaternary care

SFA   **96.** If a health care provider is caught in a fire in the health care institution, he/she should **NOT**

        A. run
        B. close all the doors and windows before leaving the area
        C. attempt to extinguish the fire if it is small
        D. call the assigned fire number

HHB   **97.** Interpretation of a quality control chart is based on the fact that for a normal distribution,

        A. 99% of the values are within ± 3 SD of the mean
        B. 99% of the values are within ± 2 SD of the mean
        C. 95% of the values are within ± 3 SD of the mean
        D. 95% of the values are within ± 1 SD of the mean

UBF   **98.** Creatinine clearance is determined through utilization of

        A. urine specimens
        B. pericardial fluid specimens
        C. synovial fluid specimens
        D. CSF specimens

IC   **99.** Which of the following is a pathogenic agent that causes nosocomial infections of the gastrointestinal tract?

        A. *Neisseria gonorrhoeae*
        B. *Vibrio cholerae*
        C. *Haemophilus vaginalis*
        D. *Bordetella pertussis*

SFA   **100.** For safety in the clinical laboratory, which of the following should **NOT** occur?

    A. Needles, syringes, and lancets should be disposed of in a special sturdy container

    B. Liquid waste should be discarded rapidly

    C. The specimen collection area should be disinfected periodically according to the clinical laboratory schedule

    D. The patients' specimens should be covered at all times during transportation

Practice Test Questions 4

Answers and Discussion

Page numbers refer to Garza D, Becan-McBride K: *Phlebotomy Handbook, 4th ed.* Stamford, CT, Appleton & Lange, 1996.

1. **(B)** Preferred skin puncture sites are the second, third, and fourth fingers. The most commonly used finger is the middle, or third, finger. Patients usually prefer their nondominant hand. *(p. 195)*

2. **(A)** Equipment for skin puncture on children and infants includes a disposable sterile automatic pediatric lancet device, a 70% isopropyl alcohol swab in a sterile package, and Microtainers. *(p. 238)*

3. **(B)** A false-negative blood culture is more likely to occur if iodine is not wiped from the tops of the blood culture tubes and if too little blood is used for the culture. *(p. 275)*

4. **(E)** Some of the problems to avoid in POC glucose testing include the following: specimen is collected at wrong time, reagents are outdated, wrong volume of specimen is collected, and calibrators are not properly used. *(p. 310)*

5. **(A)** *Pseudomonas aeruginosa, Streptococcus pneumoniae,* and Gram-negative bacilli are commonly identified pathogenic microorganisms that cause nosocomial infections of the ear. *(p. 346)*

6. (D) *(p. 528)*

7. (C) The Surgicutt and Simplate R are used for the bleeding-time procedure. *(pp. 267–268)*

8. (A) The physician-patient contract has the following basic elements: (1) the physician offers to provide a service to the patient, (2) the patient uses the service for disease treatment, and (3) the patient accepts and pays for the treatment. *(pp. 497–498)*

9. (C) The actual occurrence of an infection from a biohazardous specimen depends on the virulence of the infecting agent and the host's susceptibility. *(p. 371)*

10. (A) The anterior, or ventral, surface of the body is separated into the thoracic, abdominal, and pelvic cavities. *(p. 38)*

11. (B) The Unopette has a plastic reservoir containing a premeasured volume of reagent for diluting and has a disposable, self-filling diluting pipette consisting of a straight, thin-walled, uniform-bore, glass capillary tube fitted into a plastic holder. *(p. 143)*

12. (B) Human sperm and ova are defined as germ cells. *(p. 61)*

13. (A) Prior to a skin puncture procedure, the phlebotomist should prepare him- or herself emotionally for a positive patient encounter, prepare all supplies and equipment needed, and put on clean gloves. *(pp. 161–162, 195)*

14. (D) The HemoCue β-Glucose Analyzer can analyze glucose levels in arterial, capillary, or venous whole blood samples. *(p. 308)*

15. (B) Strict, or complete, isolation is required for patients with contagious diseases that may be transmitted by direct contact or by air. For example, patients with anthrax or rabies require strict, or complete, isolation. *(p. 353)*

16. (E) Health care workers who perform phlebotomy procedures are often asked to maintain the quality control and preventive maintenance records on thermometers, sphygmomanometers (blood pressure cuffs), centrifuges, and occasionally other types of laboratory instruments. *(pp. 460–461)*

17. **(A)** The health care worker who collects blood from an inpatient should introduce him- or herself, state that he/she is part of the hospital unit or laboratory staff, and inform the patient that a specimen is to be collected for a test ordered by the physician. *(p. 466)*

18. **(C)** A medical expert witness must testify about professional standards of care and be knowledgeable about medical practice patterns. *(p. 503)*

19. **(D)** Specimens being tested for cold agglutinins and cryofibrinogen require a heat block to warm them to body temperature for transportation and handling. *(p. 428)*

20. **(A)** Radiation exposure can be minimized by staying as far away from the radiation as possible, using lead shielding, and limiting the time of exposure. *(p. 387)*

21. **(C)** For the Surgicutt bleeding-time test, the blood pressure cuff must be inflated on the patient's upper arm to 40 mm Hg. *(p. 267)*

22. **(C)** The antecubital fossa area is most accessible and is chosen for venipuncture for most toddlers and children. *(p. 246)*

23. **(A)** Blood cortisol levels decrease in the afternoon to approximately one-half the morning value. *(p. 212)*

24. **(B)** A blood cell count including WBC count, RBC count, hemoglobin (Hgb), hematocrit (Hct), mean corpuscular volume (MCV), mean corpuscular hemoglobin (MCH), and mean corpuscular hemoglobin concentration (MCHC) requires whole blood collected in a purple-topped blood collection tube. *(pp. 108, 111, 115, 122)*

25. **(C)** Serum is blood without anticoagulant and will form a clot. For many laboratory tests, serum is removed from the blood clot that contains the cells. *(pp. 78–79)*

26. (D) The principal tasks of the clinical chemistry section include running toxicology and hormone assays. *(p. 22)*

27. (C) Blood culture tubes (yellow tops) are always collected first to reduce chances of contamination. The coagulation tube (light-blue top) should then be collected before the hematology tube (lavender top). *(p. 181)*

28. (C) *Osteomyelitis* is an inflammation of the bone due to bacterial infection. It can be caused by repeatedly puncturing the bone with a lancet. *(p. 200)*

29. (D) After the dorsal hand vein blood collection, pressure should be applied over the puncture site with a dry gauze sponge for 2–3 min. *(p. 248)*

30. (C) Blood specimens should be transported to the clinical laboratory for testing ideally within 45 min. but no longer than 2 hr. from the time of collection so that the serum or plasma can be separated from the blood cells. Once separated, serum may remain at room temperature, be refrigerated, be stored in a dark place, or be frozen, depending on the prescribed methodology. Serum should be covered to prevent evaporation. Evaporation will cause some constituents to become more concentrated and therefore will yield erroneous laboratory test results. *(p. 427)*

31. (B) "Nothing by mouth" means that the patient should have been fasting. *(p. 467)*

32. (B) *(p. 525)*

33. (B) ESR is the abbreviation for the term *sedimentation rate*. *(p. 119)*

34. (C) The venae cavae are the veins that return blood from the body to the heart. The superior vena cava returns blood from the head and upper body, while the inferior vena cava returns blood from the lower half of the body. *(p. 79)*

35. (B) An XX pair of chromosomes indicates that the baby will be a girl. *(p. 60)*

36. (D) The clinical chemistry section usually has a toxicology area for drug analysis. *(p. 22)*

37. (D) The B-D Microtainer tube is frequently used in the microcollection of electrolytes and general chemistry blood specimens. *(p. 142)*

38. (D) *(p. 531)*

39. (B) Cause-and-effect (Ishikawa) diagrams are used in quality improvement methodologies and are designed to identify interactions between people, methods, equipment, supplies, and/or reagents. *(p. 454)*

40. (B) If a health care provider is in an area of the health care facility where a fire starts, he/she should first pull the lever in the fire alarm box. *(p. 386)*

41. (B) Human chorionic gonadotropin (HCG) is the first detectable analyte produced in pregnancy. *(p. 324)*

42. (C) One of the many responsibilities of the technical supervisor of clinical laboratory sections is to prepare daily schedules to provide adequate coverage and effective use of personnel. *(p. 20)*

43. (C) Metabolism involves making necessary substances or breaking down chemical substances in order to use energy. *(p. 43)*

44. (C) A differential count enumerates percentages of specific leukocytes in the blood. It is usually performed in a hematology laboratory. *(p. 88)*

45. (A) The hepatic artery delivers blood to the liver. (*See* color atlas.)

46. (D) *(p. 525)*

47. (C) Disinfectants are chemical compounds used to remove or kill pathogenic microorganisms. *(pp. 372–373)*

48. (B) Pericardial fluid is collected from the sac around the heart. *(p. 330)*

49. (A) The Unopette is a blood collection device prefilled with specific amounts of diluents or reagents. *(p. 143)*

50. (D) Individuals with type O blood are called *universal donors.* *(p. 76)*

51. (A) Normal humans have 2 lungs. The left lung has only 2 lobes, whereas the right lung has 3 lobes. *(p. 54)*

52. (D) The Autolet II Clinisafe is a spring-activated puncture device with three disposable platforms for control of penetration depth. *(p. 138)*

53. (C) The direct Coomb's test is performed in the immunohematology section. *(pp. 27–28)*

54. (B) Blood cholesterol levels increase with age. *(p. 212)*

55. (A) The photograph shows Samplette capillary blood collectors. *(p. 141)*

56. (B) To obtain the blood trough level for a medication, the patient's blood should be collected immediately prior to the administration of the medication. *(p. 284)*

57. (C) A random urine sample is the specimen of choice for a urinary pregnancy test. *(p. 324)*

58. (B) Tolerance limits for a quality control chart are determined by pooling the data obtained during a 20-day test period and referring to the mean ±2 standard deviations. *(p. 310)*

59. (B) Falsely increased values of a blood analyte can be mistakenly interpreted as elevated or normal if the blood analyte is truly in a normal range or a decreased range, respectively. *(p. 214)*

60. (C) The containers in Figure 4-2 are needle-disposal containers (Datar, Inc.) for disposal of used needles and sharps to reduce the possibility of needlestick injuries. *(p. 130)*

61. (D) Avoiding the use of gloves with talc powder when collecting blood is recommended because the tubes of patients' blood may become contaminated with this powder and result in falsely elevated calcium values. *(p. 135)*

62. (A) With therapeutic drug monitoring, the physician must know the time and date of collection, whether the blood was collected before or after drug administration, and in some cases, the length of infusion time. *(p. 468)*

63. (E) The medical record allows for continuity of the patient's care plan, documents the patient's illness and treatment, documents communication between the physician and other members of the health care team, and provides a legal document for patients, the hospital, and employees. *(pp. 504–505)*

64. (E) Labeled skin puncture specimens should include the patient's name and identification number, time of collection, phlebotomist's initials, and date of collection. Preparation, identification, and handling should be the same for skin puncture specimens as for venipuncture specimens. *(p. 184, 195)*

65. (E) Reasons for not using arm veins are the following: The patient has IV lines in both arms, is burned, has casts on both arms, has thrombosed veins, or has edematous arms. *(pp. 167, 169)*

66. (E) Specimens for zinc, transaminase, testosterone, and rubella determinations are all collected in speckled-topped blood collection tubes to obtain serum *(pp. 119, 120)*

67. (B) Tests for blood typing and donor cross-match testing are performed in an immunohematology, a transfusion, or a blood banking laboratory. *(p. 88)*

68. (B) The digestive system functions, first, to break down food chemically and physically into nutrients that can be absorbed and used by body cells, and second, to eliminate the waste products of digestion. *(p. 56)*

69. (C) Violent crying and medications can falsely alter laboratory test results dramatically. *(pp. 211–212, 213–214)*

70. (E) Hyperthyroidism, pregnancy, adrenal insufficiency, and acute pancreatitis are conditions that may affect the results of the GTT. *(p. 280)*

71. (E) Basic responsibilities of health care managers or supervisors include all of the following: evaluating technical performance, measuring turnaround times, monitoring the budget and expenses, and scheduling work hours. *(pp. 485–487)*

72. (E) Characteristics of malpractice cases typically include (1) the plaintiff believes that the health care provider did something wrong, (2) the plaintiff was injured, (3) the health care provider failed to use professional standards of care, and (4) damage was physical, emotional, or financial. *(pp. 495, 496)*

73. (E) The human body has distinctive characteristics: a backbone, bisymmetry, body cavities, and 11 major organ systems. *(p. 38)*

74. (D) Gray-topped blood collection tubes can be ordered containing potassium oxalate and sodium fluoride. *(p. 108)*

75. (B) The sagittal plane runs lengthwise and divides the body into right and left halves. *(p. 38)*

76. (E) For determinations of ammonia levels, chromosome analysis, determinations of cryofibrinogen levels, and the LE cell test, blood must be collected in green-topped blood collection tubes. *(pp. 109, 112, 113, 116)*

77. (D) When arm veins cannot be used, veins in the posterior surface (dorsal side) of the wrist are preferred over ankle or foot veins because the lower extremities tend to have more frequent coagulation and vascular complications than the upper extremities do. The anterior (ventral) side of the wrist should *not* be used because of the numerous tendons present and nerve sensitivity in this area. *(p. 169)*

78. **(A)** Swollen fingers, excessive milking of the finger, and using the first drop of blood all have an adverse effect on the quality of a finger stick. *(pp. 195, 200)*

79. **(C)** Forcing blood into an evacuated collection tube from a syringe and vigorously shaking the specimen tube are two ways to cause hemolysis of the specimen. *(p. 209)*

80. **(C)** Figure 4-3 shows swabbing of the arm in concentric circles in preparation of collecting blood for blood cultures or blood donations. *(pp. 272, 292)*

81. **(A)** The nose, trachea, and lungs are all components of the respiratory system. *(p. 53)*

82. **(A)** The volume of plasma or serum that can generally be collected from a premature infant is approximately 100–150 uL, and about two times that amount can be collected from a full-term newborn. Larger volumes are obtained from older children and adults. *(p. 137)*

83. **(E)** The label on the blood specimen or body fluid specimen must include the patient's name, the patient's identification number, the time at which the specimen is collected, the attending physician's name, the date, and the type of specimen. *(pp. 158, 184)*

84. **(C)** The ankles, wrists, and toes are not suitable sites for skin puncture. *(p. 195)*

85. **(A)** If the needle is inserted through the vein, the vacuum in the specimen tube is lost, or the patient's veins are sclerosed, the phlebotomist may fail to collect blood. *(pp. 205, 208)*

86. **(A)** Falsely low levels of lidocaine, phenytoin, and pentobarbital occur with the use of gel serum separator tubes. *(p. 285)*

87. **(E)** Infection control logs and reports, JCAHO standards, laboratory policies and procedures, and board certification are all part of "discovery" in a blood collection lawsuit. *(p. 502)*

88. **(B)** Staffing for phlebotomy services involves recruitment, selection, placement, training, development through continuing education, scheduling, compensation, and evaluation of employees' productivity and performance. *(p. 486)*

89. **(A)** Westgard and his colleagues suggest a "5 Q" framework for clinical laboratories that focuses on quality planning, quality laboratory practices, quality control of processes, quality assessment (performance monitoring), and quality improvement when problems occur. *(pp. 454–455)*

90. **(A)** Computer transmission devices can provide on-line reporting systems and are more reliable than verbal reports. Verbal reports are acceptable, but they are subject to errors. Facsimile (fax) reports are acceptable if they are being received by the appropriate individuals. *(p. 433)*

91. **(E)** A laboratory-acquired infection can result from (1) drinking or eating in the specimen collection area, (2) popping the cap off a vacuum collection tube, (3) sustaining scratches from needles, and (4) rubbing the eyes in the specimen collection area. *(p. 371)*

92. **(B)** The glucose tolerance test (GTT) requires numerous blood collections. *(pp. 276, 281)*

93. **(D)** The carotid arteries provide blood to the head and neck regions of the body. *(See* color atlas.)

94. **(D)** Glycogen is the form of stored glucose in muscles. Exercise increases the amount of glycogen available for muscles. *(p. 51)*

95. **(A)** Primary care is given to maintain and monitor normal health and to prevent diseases through immunizations. *(p. 7)*

96. (A) If a health care provider is caught in a fire in the health care institution, he/she should **NOT** run. *(p. 386)*

97. (A) For a normal distribution, 99% of the control values are within ± 3SD of the mean. *(p. 310)*

98. (A) The creatinine clearance is determined through utilization of urine and blood specimens. *(p. 323)*

99. (B) *Vibrio cholerae* is a pathogenic agent that causes nosocomial infections of the gastrointestinal tract. *(p. 346)*

100. (B) Liquid waste must be disposed of gently so that the liquid does not splash onto other objects. *(pp. 381–382)*

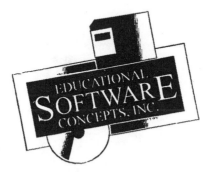

Installation Instructions

1. Put disk in drive.
2. Click START. (If you have Windows 3.x, from Program Manager click FILE.)
3. Click RUN.
4. Type A:\setup and press ENTER.
5. Follow the on-screen instructions.

If you are having problems installing or running our software, please call ESC, Inc. at (800) 748-7734.